DISEASE CHANGE AND THE ROLE OF MEDICINE

Comparative Studies of Health Systems and Medical Care

General Editor
CHARLES LESLIE

Editorial Board
FRED DUNN, M.D., University of California, San Francisco
RENÉE FOX, University of Pennsylvania
ELIOT FREIDSON, New York University
EWARD MONTGOMERY, Washington University
YASUO OTSUKA, M.D., Yokohama City University Medical School
CARL E. TAYLOR, M.D., The Johns Hopkins University
K. N. UDUPA, M.S., F.R.C.S., Banaras Hindu University
PAUL UNSCHULD, University of Marburg

John M. Janzen, *The Quest for Therapy in Lower Zaire*
Paul V. Unschuld, *Medical Ethics in Imperial China: A Study in Historical Anthropology*
Margaret M. Lock, *East Asian Medicine in Urban Japan: Varieties of Medical Experience*
Jeanie Schmit Kayser-Jones, *Old, Alone, and Neglected: Care of the Aged in Scotland and in the United States*
Arthur Kleinman, *Patients and Healers in the Context of Culture: An Exploration of the Borderland Between Anthropology, Medicine and Psychiatry*
Stephen J. Kunitz, *Disease Change and the Role of Medicine: The Navajo Experience*

Disease Change and the Role of Medicine: The Navajo Experience

Stephen J. Kunitz

University of California Press, Berkeley, Los Angeles, London

University of California Press
Berkeley and Los Angeles, California

University of California Press, Ltd.
London, England
First paperback printing 1989
Copyright © 1983 by The Regents of the University of California

Library of Congress Cataloging in Publication Data

Kunitz, Stephen J.
  Disease change and the role of medicine.

  (Comparative studies of health systems and medical care)
  Includes index.
  1. Navajo Indians—Diseases. 2. Navajo Indians—Mortality. 3. Navajo
Indians—Medical care. 4. Navajo Indians—Medicine. 5. Indians of
North America—Southwest, New—Diseases. 6. Indians of North America—
Southwest, New—Mortality. 7. Indians of North America—Southwest,
New—Medical care. 8. Indians of North

  ISBN 0-520-06789-4

Printed in the United States of America

1 2 3 4 5 6 7 8 9

For Lisa and Daniel

May their love for America and Americans be ever broad enough to embrace all lands and peoples struggling for the good life.

Contents

Acknowledgments

NUMEROUS friends and colleagues have helped with various aspects of this work, and it is with pleasure that I acknowledge their assistance. Much of the early data collection was done with the financial support of grant GI-34837 from the National Science Foundation. That was my piece of a large study called the Lake Powell Research Project which brought together in an unlikely consortium investigators from many disciplines and several universities across the country. I am grateful to all my colleagues on the project with whom I shared much bourbon, scotch, and stimulating conversation. I am particularly grateful to Orson Anderson, who originated the study, and to Priscilla Grew who was the executive secretary. My debt to Jerrold Levy, who was coordinator of the social science projects and has been both a friend and collaborator before and since, is especially great.

My work would not have been possible without the help of many people in the Indian Health Service of the U.S. Public Health Service: David Broudy, Marlene Haffner, Aaron Handler, Edward Helmick, Bill McGovern, and Mozart Spector. In addition, a contract from the Navajo Area Office of the Indian Health Service (No. 245-78-0187) provided helpful support in the later phases of data analysis.

John C. Slocumb, a friend since we were medical students and a colleague and collaborator since then, first interested me in demography. I am grateful to him for allowing me to include as part of chapter 3 material first published in an article we wrote together on maternal morbidity and mortality. Charles L.

Odoroff and K. Reuben Gabriel have provided invaluable statistical advice and consolation. Kurt Deuschle many years ago encouraged my interest in working as a physician on the Navajo Reservation and more recently has commented upon sections of the manuscript. David Aberle has influenced many of my ideas and as the not-so-anonymous reviewer of the manuscript for the University of California Press has made many very helpful suggestions. Helena Temkin-Greener did much of the data analysis while working with me as a postdoctoral fellow supported by grant 1F 32 HD-5806-01 from the National Institute of Child Health and Human Development. Charles Leslie has been a ruthless and always supportive editor.

Some of the material presented in the book was first published elsewhere. Chapter 1 is a slightly revised version of a paper that first appeared in *Human Biology*. Some of the material in chapters 2 and 3 also appeared first in *Human Biology* and in *Human Organization*. I am grateful to the editors of each journal for permission to use it here. Chapter 4 is based upon material first published in *Ethnicity and Medical Care*, edited by Alan Harwood. It is used here with the permission of Harvard University Press.

It is customary at this point in the acknowledgments for the author to absolve all his advisors of any responsibility for mistakes and to thank his family for their support through a very trying time. I shall depart from that tradition first by saying that if so many smart friends and colleagues have not been able to save me from myself, they carry as large a share of the responsibility as I do, if not larger. I would have listened if they would have only said something. Second, writing this book has been fun. My wife Izzie and our children Lisa and Daniel made it more fun, even when the latter two wondered out loud why they were being schlepped to England so their father could write a book about America.

Introduction

BEGINNING in the seventeenth century in Western Europe and later elsewhere, human population began to grow at an unprecedentedly high and sustained rate. Though increased fertility has been implicated as one of the contributing causes, a continuous dramatic fall in mortality has been of at least equal and probably greater significance. The decline in mortality—what has been termed the epidemiological transition (Omran 1971)—has been the result of a decline in pandemics and epidemics of infectious diseases. As they have waned, man-made and degenerative diseases, often with a very significant psychosocial component to their etiology (Cassel 1970, 1974), have become relatively more important in contributing to mortality.

The cause of the decline in infectious diseases has been a matter of debate. Some have attributed the decline to improved living conditions—such as improved sanitation, better housing, and more adequate diets—while others have claimed that medical measures have been largely responsible. The latter I shall term the *heroic history* of medicine; the former the *revisionist history*. In recent years the revisionist version has gained considerably in popularity. The differences between them may be accounted for largely by the populations examined and the length of the periods considered.

For example, McKeown (1976*a*, 1976*b*) as well as others have shown that in Northwestern Europe and the United States, the dramatic declines in mortality that occurred during the nineteenth century antedated the introduction of specific therapies. Moreover, medicine's contribution, though real, accounted for only a small proportion of the decline that took place during the twentieth century. A series of impressive graphs in McKeown's (1976*a*) book illustrate this point, each one showing the decline in death rate from a particular disease over a century or more with an arrow placed at the date when a specific therapy was introduced. Almost invariably, most of the decline had happened before the crucial date.

The heroic version, often espoused by highly placed biomedical researchers, claims the conquest of infectious disease was related to advances made by modern medicine (Seldin 1975, 1976). These accounts often consider only the period after the introduction of antimicrobial therapy in the United States and Western Europe and show that indeed the therapy was effective in diminishing the mortality rate.

Many workers in public health and related fields find the debate surprising. They have always "known" that social conditions influence mortality and that improvements in the former are causally related to declines in the latter. They have also believed—though with varying degrees of intensity—that curative medicine has had an important role to play, particularly in Third World populations. The debate, however, suggests that there is not nearly as much agreement as many of us have assumed on the contribution medicine has made to improved health of different populations. Moreover, these different historical interpretations are neither arcane nor trivial but have very real implications for health care and research policy. The heroic view assumes that the triumphs of the past will be repeated with a new class of diseases in the future. Just as infectious diseases were conquered, so will those of a degenerative and man-made nature be vanquished by more biomedical research and its application to individual patients. With such a promise, it is difficult to resist pouring ever increasing amounts of money into wars on cancer and other killers of emerging or established importance.

By contrast, the revisionist view suggests that environmental and social determinants ("life-style") are especially important. The result in terms of policy is support of a variety of preventive efforts—such as improved dietary patterns and reduction in smoking—and less support for curative medicine as practiced by individual physicians. No wonder, then, that the revisionist view has struck such a responsive chord among health planners. It goes a long way toward rationalizing efforts for cost containment in an inflationary period and, not incidentally, provides ammunition with which these low-status professionals may attack those of greater eminence.

It should be clear that there is much in the revisionist view that I accept, notably that in the industrialized nations of Western Europe and North America the major decline in mortality antedated the development of specific medical therapies (Kunitz, in press). Indeed, both mortality decline and the emergence of medicine as we know it, beginning in the latter half of the nineteenth century, were the effects of a common cause, the transformations wrought by industrial capitalism. I believe, however, that to generalize the revisionist interpretation to other populations may have unintended but pernicious consequences. That is to say, it may rationalize the withholding of therapy that does work from those populations that may benefit from it, notably those of the Third World and the poor within the developed nations.

There is another point of importance. If evidence shows that specific therapies have reduced mortality and morbidity from infectious diseases, are we justified in assuming, as historians of the heroic persuasion do, that the same will be the case with the noninfectious degenerative and man-made diseases? Similarly, if we believe that medical therapy has been of very little significance, should we assume, as revisionist historians do, that it will be of little value in treating diseases of increasing importance? It may well be the case that success—or lack of it—in treating infectious diseases will be replicated only imperfectly or not at all in the treatment of degenerative and man-made diseases.

Indeed, the argument I shall present in this book is that among Navajo Indians, an undisputably poor population in a generally wealthy society, medical therapy was of enormous value in treating some of the most important infectious diseases but is and will continue to be of questionable value in reducing mortality from the causes that are now of major significance— accidental and other violent deaths. If this is so, then it is important to ask, what role modern medicine does play? The answer, I suggest, is that increasingly medicine acts as an acculturating agent, teaching people to define conditions that are largely psychosocial in origin and rooted in traditional patterns of ecological adaptation and social organization as diseases for which new modes of explanation, treatment, and behavior are necessary.

This position is somewhat different from that of Trowell and Burkitt (1981), who in their recent book on *Western Diseases: Their Emergence and Prevention* specifically exempt from consideration such important conditions as accidents and other forms of violence while at the same time defining Western diseases as "essentially the 'man-made diseases' " (p. xiv). What they do include, various forms of cancer and certain gastrointestinal, metabolic, and cardiovascular diseases, are more obviously organic than the causes of death they exclude. Thus their chapter on North American Indians does not include a consideration of accidents, the single most frequent cause of death in that population and clearly of greater significance now than several decades ago. This neglect is very likely because they are made uncomfortable by calling accidents and violence diseases. I share that discomfort, and part of my book is devoted to considering what it means when a society defines conditions as diseases instead of something else. Nonetheless, however one defines particular conditions, if they account for many deaths and are of new and growing importance, they cannot simply be ignored but must be considered and, if possible, explained.

This book is organized in the following fashion. Chapter 1 provides comparative data on contemporary mortality rates and patterns among several different American Indian tribes, including the Navajos, for two purposes: first, to set the Navajos within a larger context; and second, to make the point that the most important causes of mortality as well as total mortality do not vary randomly but are ranked depending upon the tribes' traditional patterns of ecological adaptation prior to the reservation period. As the epidemic infectious diseases have waned and diseases that are more psychosocial in origin have become of relatively increased importance, variations in mortality rates have become discernible that reflect the degree to which tribes were more or less prepared for, or preadapted to, the reservation situation. Sedentary agriculturalists with already developed mechanisms of social control rooted in the hierarchical nature of their society were better suited for life on reservations than were the former hunter-gatherers whose means of conflict resolution traditionally involved dispersion, a mechanism no longer possible in the present setting. Navajos, who were pastoralists, are intermediate between these two groups.

Chapter 2 is an economic and demographic history of the Navajo reservation from the late nineteenth century to the present. The Navajos are the largest Indian tribe in North America, numbering approximately 150,000 on a reservation of 24,000 square miles, with perhaps another 20,000 to 30,000 living away from the reservation. The reservation, located in Arizona, New Mexico, and Utah, contains oil, coal, and uranium. Despite the richness of their natural resources, the Navajos have a per capita income of about 25 percent of the national average. The epidemiologic and demographic consequences of their history of economic nondevelopment are the focus of discussion in this chapter. The points made are, first, that economic nondevelopment makes the extended kin network an appropriate adaptation to the contemporary scene at the same time as it discourages the use of family planning; second, regional variations have existed among areas of the reservation for at least sixty years and probably longer and are now reflected in dependence upon welfare and occasional wage work in some places or wage work alone in others; third, the relatively employable young move from the former to the latter areas, leaving behind a residual population of the elderly and the less employable. While age-specific fertility rates are higher in the poorer areas, mortality rates are generally low throughout the reservation at present. Thus, the rate of natural increase is higher in the poorer areas than elsewhere. And fourth, there is evidence, discussed further in chapter 3, that mortality increased in the early decades of the twentieth century and began to decrease beginning in the 1940s.

Chapter 3 traces the history of several causes of death over the past century and shows that for tuberculosis and maternal mortality, medical interventions were of major significance in reducing mortality, even in the face of minimal economic change. Reductions in infant mortality, by contrast, were apparently related to improvements in nutrition and sanitation. Accidents and violence have increased and are most common among young adult males. Analyses by region show that accidents are the most important cause of variation in crude mortality rates and are highest in areas where the population is most dependent upon wage work; furthermore, the high rates are largely due to the influx of young adults who seek employment in these areas.

Chapter 4 describes traditional Navajo beliefs regarding disease causation, patterns of utilization of traditional healers, and changes from Navajo religion to peyotism and Christianity. A decline in the number of singers is attributed to the expense of training and to the fact that potential apprentices leave home to search for work. The sings that are performed are often short versions of longer and more expensive ceremonies. These changes are largely due to a decline in the livestock economy. By contrast, the core values of Navajo religion, largely focused upon individual health and well-being, have not changed. Finally, the use of Western medicine is not necessarily antithetical to traditional Navajo beliefs, which were focused upon cure rather than symptomatic relief. The use of physicians, like the use of herbalists, to provide symptomatic relief may be pursued along with traditional curing ceremonies. The real decline in Navajo religious practice, then, has not been caused primarily by proselytizing Western physicians but by other more profound social and economic forces. Medical workers, however, have played a role in this change.

Chapter 5 describes changes in the use of hospitals and clinics since the 1920s. The utilization of hospitals increased rapidly during the 1920s and 1930s as the number of beds increased. A sharp decline between 1940 and 1955 was due to the diversion of medical resources to the military during World War II and to changes in federal Indian policy, which reduced the number of beds and staff. A rapid increase in utilization from 1955 to the late 1960s followed a reversal in policy that again increased facilities. Throughout the 1970s the number of hospital admissions remained essentially constant, but change in morbidity caused a decline in pediatric admissions and a slow increase in admissions of the elderly. Thus the social role of the hospital changed as disease patterns changed. Nonemergent conditions assume relatively greater significance as emergent conditions decline. For example, the highest proportion of elderly patients currently come from wage work communities where families are not prepared to care for them at home. And an analysis of gynecological procedures that are as technically complex but less urgent than other surgical procedures shows that they are used by people from wage-work communities to terminate or avoid childbearing and to alleviate symptoms that more traditional women regard as inevitable. The point is that the social determinants of utilization change as admissions become increasingly discretionary.

Chapter 6 argues that as the health care system increasingly confronts problems such as alcohol abuse and automobile accidents, the socialization function of medicine assumes greater importance and the medical role increasingly becomes one of defining a variety of social conditions as health problems. Since the newly important problems are related to patterns of social organization rooted in ecological adaptations made centuries ago, they are likely to be especially refractory to medical interventions. By encouraging the Navajos to use the definitions of health care professionals, medicine increasingly assumes an acculturating role.

The results have implications beyond the Navajos, for along with other recent studies (e.g., Preston 1976; Berggren et al. 1981) they show that medical therapy has been effective in some important instances in less developed nations and in segments of the populations of developed ones. They also suggest, however, that the triumphs of the past may not be predictive of equal success in the future, as new causes of morbidity and mortality emerge which are diverse in origin and for which there is no explanatory theory as inclusive and powerful as the germ theory. In the absence of such a unifying paradigm (Lower and Kanarek 1982), the medical profession is increasingly subject to attack from without and segementation from within. One response among segments of the profession as well as the lay public is to expand the concept of disease to encompass all manner of human distress. It is this redefinition of many conditions as diseases that we see increasingly at work among Navajos as well as many other populations.

1

Mortality, Fertility, and Social Organization

EPIDEMIC infectious diseases are relatively recent phenomena in human history. For most of man's time on earth, populations were small, scattered, and dependent upon hunting and gathering. Those infectious diseases that affected humans were either the result of accidental infection by zoonoses or indolent infections that perhaps had evolved with humans from their primate ancestors. It was only as a result of the agricultural revolution 6,000 to 8,000 years ago and the consequent growth of sedentary populations large enough to support microorganisms specifically dependent upon human hosts that epidemics appear to have become part of man's life (Cockburn 1963; Black 1966, 1975).

The result of the emergence of epidemics was that mortality became an increasingly significant determinant of population growth. This was because there is a limit to how many children a woman can bear but no limit to mortality except total extinction. It was only in the seventeenth and eighteenth centuries in Western Europe that epidemics began to wane and population began to increase dramatically. There is reason to believe that increased fertility contributed substantially to the growth of population, but there is no doubt that a major contribution was the decline in mortality (Habakkuk 1971).

While population began to grow in Europe, in the New World there were devastating losses as new epidemic diseases were introduced by Europeans into the Indian population.

Smallpox, measles, and other infectious diseases led to the loss of millions of lives in the years after first contact, and high rates of death from these causes persisted into the present century (Dobyns 1966, 1976).

In the meantime, in Europe and among the colonists in the New World, epidemics continued to wane in significance so that ultimately the Age of Pestilence and Famine gave way to the Age of Receding Pandemics, which in turn gave way to the Age of Man-Made and Degenerative Diseases (Omran 1971, 1977). In this last period, mortality rates have become so low that fertility has become the major determinant of population growth.

Among underdeveloped nations, the transition from one stage of disease to another began later but has been much more rapid because of the importation of various techniques of death control, such as public health measures, curative medicine, and the like. This has been true for Indians in North America as well as for other colonial peoples. The result has been the recent emergence of some of the same new causes of morbidity and mortality that affect the larger society—man-made and degenerative diseases, the etiology of which includes psychosocial factors to a greater degree than is likely to have been the case with the epidemic infectious diseases. The increased significance of psychosocial factors affects even the infectious diseases, many of which are now caused not by extrinsic organisms but by those that live in constant association with humans and only cause illness when the host experiences some sort of stress.

Based upon a review of many epidemiological and laboratory animal studies, Cassel (1974) has suggested that most significant among these psychosocial factors are membership in a group, status within the group, and preparedness for a new situation. The precise mechanism through which these factors operate is not clear, though it is probably related to the pituitary-adrenal axis (Selye 1956). It does not seem likely, however, that the workings of the neuroendocrine system best explain such phenomena as homicides, suicides, and accidents. Nonetheless, the concept of preparedness for a new situation will prove useful when I discuss these phenomena.

Much of the human race is entering or has already entered the age of man-made and degenerative diseases. Thus concern with host factors of a psychosocial nature has grown. Enhancing that concern is the notion held by many social scientists that social change and acculturation are accompanied by many dysfunctional consequences, including pathological behavior and stress-related diseases. Too often, however, the consequences of social change have been seen as determined by the dominant society rather than as produced by the interaction between a subordinate society with a history, culture, and social organization of its own and a larger society to which it is acculturating.

In the case of American Indians, for instance, one sometimes gets the impression from what has been written that virtually all tribes have responded in essentially the same fashion to increasing contact with Anglo-Americans and their institutions. Such contact seems to be inevitably attended by social disorganization, heavy drinking, homicides, accidental deaths, and a variety of other forms of destructive and self-destructive behavior. Previous work, however, has suggested that tribes differ in the incidence, prevalence, and patterns of these various behaviors and that these differences are related in a consistent way to traditional forms of social organization as they existed in the prereservation period (Levy and Kunitz 1974). Briefly, band-level tribes were found to have higher rates of homicide and suicide than pastoralists, and pastoralists in turn had higher rates than sedentary agriculturalists. These differences, as well as differences in patterns of alcohol use, appeared to be related to differing mechanisms of social control in populations with varying types of ecological adaptation.

Savishinsky (1971) has observed that when tribes whose primary mode of ecological adaptation has involved considerable dispersion and movement come together in larger groups, conflicts are generated for which an important means of resolution is dispersion. As he puts it, "When high mobility is a basic feature of a society's ecology, then movement will also be utilized by the people as a way to relieve social sources of stress" (Savishinsky 1971:615).

By contrast, among sedentary people dispersion is a means of social control used only as a last resort. Hopis, for instance, have used village splitting or ejection of deviant individuals as a means of control but usually after other means, such as gossip, lecturing, witchcraft accusations, and mocking by clowns at public dances, have failed.

Finally, sedentary tribes tend to be more socially stratified than egalitarian bands of hunter-gatherers. Statuses are more likely to be inherited among the former than among the latter, for whom individual achievement was a more realistic possibility.

Based upon these observations, it was hypothesized that members of American Indian tribes in which social control and stratification were well developed in the prereservation period would likely be better prepared for life as subordinate members of a colonial society than would members of tribes that were originally egalitarian and dependent largely upon dispersion for ameliorating stress and conflict. If that is the case, then it would be expected that tribes that were originally loosely organized in hunting-gathering bands would not only have higher death rates from homicides, accidents, and suicides than would sedentary agricultural tribes, but also would have higher crude death rates as well. As Cassel (1970:198) suggests, "Social factors may increase the risk of ill health by increasing *general susceptibility* to disease" (emphasis added). Semisedentary tribes would be expected to be intermediate between these two extremes.

Fertility is generally said to follow mortality in the transition process. That is, as mortality declines it seems to be the case that fertility also declines, but at varying rates. It would thus be expected that tribes with higher mortality rates would also have higher fertility rates. A complicating feature, however, is that fertility control is dependent to some considerable degree on the ability to use contraception and this, in turn, may be dependent on personality structure, particularly on the degree to which individuals are impulsive in their behavior. If personality structure varies consistently with social organization, and if mortality does also, then disentangling the relative contributions of mortality rates and personality to fertility would be difficult at best.

Very little is known of aboriginal patterns of fertility in tribes with different types of social organization and economic subsistence. Some investigators have suggested that agriculturalists with an assured food supply would likely develop pronatalist beliefs. Conversely, hunters without an assured supply would be more sensitive to a fluctuating resource base and would be more likely to limit their population in a variety of ways. With a few exceptions (Lee 1972), data are not readily available for such comparative studies. Such data would be most likely found in populations where vital statistics are kept, and these are almost by definition populations in which contact with a colonizing society has been established and where epidemic disease, medical care, and economic exploitation have already been introduced (Polgar 1972). In general, it seems to be the case that for Southwestern American Indian tribes with a variety of types of social organization, fertility was generally high in the early reservation period (late nineteenth and twentieth centuries).

Most studies of acculturation have been concerned with the contact situation, whether it is directive or nondirective (Spicer 1961). There is less consistent concern with the ways in which societies with different types of social organization respond to the contact situation. In the present instance, it is assumed that the situation for all tribes was essentially the same: coercive and aimed at changing the subordinate Indian societies in ways deemed desirable by the dominant society. The fact that all the tribes discussed in this chapter are on reservations indicates that to a certain degree this is the case. The size and location of reservations and populations are themselves critical factors, leading to greater or lesser isolation from day-to-day contact with the agents and institutions of the dominant society. The Navajos are perhaps the most isolated tribe in this regard and the Eastern Pueblos perhaps the least, though Shoshone-Bannocks have also had much contact with local Anglo-Americans (J. G. Jorgensen, personal communication). In this analysis, however, it must be assumed that the differences are not as significant as the similarities.

Even though American Indians in the Southwest and Rocky Mountain West have been on reservations and the recipients of federal programs since the latter half of the nineteenth century, the population data, vital statistics, and economic information that are uniformly collected and published have been of generally poor quality. This must be emphasized because any conclusions drawn from these data are to be regarded as more suggestive than definitive. The sources are all published material collected for administrative and planning rather than research purposes. The rigor and uniformity with which they were gathered is therefore unknown. It is assumed here, however, that whatever errors exist are randomly distributed and that there are no consistent biases in over- or underreporting, except for a few that are mentioned below.

In the mid-1950s, the United States Public Health Service (USPHS) took over the health care of American Indians from the Bureau of Indian Affairs and published a volume on Indian health (USPHS 1957), which included information on age-specific death rates, causes of death, a variety of measures of fertility, and so on. The information came from state health departments and the Bureau of the Census as well as from special surveys carried out by the USPHS itself. As in subsequent PHS publications, it is not clear how tribal membership of individuals was determined nor how accurately the populations of the various reservations were enumerated. Presumably there was somewhat greater accuracy on all counts among the smaller tribes as opposed to those among the Navajos, the largest American Indian tribe. These data are displayed in table 1.1.

TABLE 1.1
BIRTH AND DEATH RATES, 1949–1953 AVERAGED

Agency or reservation	Tribe(s)*	Birth rate per 1,000 women, 15–44	Age-adjusted death rate	Age-specific death rate < 1 yr.
Nevada	Paiute	166	15.2	81
Fort Hall	Shoshone-Bannock	202	15.7	84
Western Apache	White Mt. & San Carlos Apaches	195	17.4	154
Mescalero	Mescalero Apaches (Eastern)	215.4	15.0	–
Pine Ridge	Sioux	153.3	11.3	60.8
Rosebud	Sioux	195.7	14.5	89.0
Pima-Papago	Pima-Papago	137	12.0	115
United Pueblo	Eastern Pueblos	146	10.5	97

Source: USPHS 1957

*Navajos and Hopis omitted because they were combined in the original publication.

A second source of data is publications from the Public Health Service for calendar years 1968 and 1969, which provide information on fertility and mortality in different service units (USPHS 1970*a*, 1970*b*). These service units are geographic regions in which care is provided by the PHS. It is often unclear what the units' boundaries are, what the actual resident population is, and what the tribal membership of residents is. Thus, if a death certificate of an Indian living in the Keams Canyon Service Unit is found, it is most likely that of a Hopi Indian but may in fact be that of a Navajo living in the Joint Use Area. In general, service units chosen for analysis are those for which there is a reasonable degree of certainty that the vast majority of residents were of one tribe and for which 1970 census data were available to provide a population denominator for the calculation of rates. These data refer not to all members of a tribe but only to those living on the reservation.

The census itself is problematic, particularly for the Navajos (U.S. Bureau of the Census 1973), for there is a wide discrepancy between estimates of reservation resident population from the Bureau of Indian Affairs (BIA) (130,000 plus or minus 10 percent in 1972) and those from the U.S. Census (about 60,000 in 1970) (U.S. Bureau of the Census 1972). For this study, BIA data were adjusted downward to estimate 1970 levels, though in all other cases census counts have been used.

Census data concerning education, income, and employment are not available from all reservations. Information is provided for those reservations where it is available. A second source of employment data is the BIA (U.S. Bureau of Indian Affairs 1973), whose data are *estimates* of the size of the labor force and the number of individuals employed, unemployed, and underemployed. As these data are estimates provided by individuals knowledgeable about each tribe, they are about the best available. Nonetheless, it must be kept in mind that they are estimates.

Though there are many deficiencies in the information available, there are some attractive features that make it worthwhile. First, I know of no other place in the world where it is possible to compare tribes with different types of social organization for which the data are any better. Second, the accessibility and quality of medical care provided to each tribe are essentially the same. In each case there are hospitals and clinics staffed by the Indian

Health Service of the U.S. Public Health Service where care is given free of charge. Third, vis-à-vis the dominant society, each tribe is an ethnic minority facing somewhat similar problems in terms of the quality of education provided, access to wage work, and racial discrimination.

Data concerning social organization come from Murdock's (1967) ethnographic atlas. The variables were chosen to give an indication of: (1) the relative importance of various sources of subsistence; and (2) the mobility of the population and patterns of settlement.

Settlement is defined as seminomadic, semisedentary, and sedentary. Seminomadic means that members wander in bands but occupy a fixed settlement at some season(s) of the year. Semisedentary means that the population moves from one fixed settlement to another at different seasons of the year. Sedentary means that the population resides in permanent villages. Subsistence refers to the relative degree of dependence various populations had upon hunting and/or gathering, agriculture, and, in the postcontact period, animal husbandry.

The tribes are the following: Shoshone-Bannocks, Eastern Apaches (Mescalero and Jicarilla); Western Apaches (San Carlos and White Mountain); Navajos; Hopis; Pimas; Papagos; Paiutes; and the Eastern Pueblos of Nambe, San Juan, Cochiti, San Ildefonso, Santa Clara, Tesque, Pojoaque, Santo Domingo, and San Felipe (all of which are in the Santa Fe Service Unit); and the Rosebud and Pine Ridge Sioux.

The summary data from Murdock's (1967) atlas refer to the postcontact period and are as follows: the Paiutes and Shoshone-Bannocks were seminomadic and dependent on hunting and gathering; the Western Apaches were semisedentary and dependent on hunting, gathering, and agriculture to about equal degrees; the Navajos, though also semisedentary, were more dependent on animal husbandry than were the other western Apaches. The Navajos and the White Mountain Apaches were heavily influenced by the Pueblos, particularly after the revolt against the Spanish in 1680, and much of this influence is evident in their ceremonial structure (Underhill 1948). The Eastern Apaches are classified as seminomadic and dependent primarily on hunting and gathering; the Papagos were semisedentary and dependent primarily on agriculture; the Pimas, Eastern Pueblos, and Hopis (the westernmost Pueblo tribe) were sedentary and almost exclusively dependent on agriculture, whereas the Sioux were seminomadic and dependent primarily on hunting.

The data for 1968–69 are displayed in Table 1.2 and have been analyzed by use of the biplot (Gabriel 1971, 1973; Gabriel et al. 1974). Since this technique may not be familiar to many readers and will be used in subsequent chapters as well, I will describe briefly how to interpret the figures, reserving for the next section an analysis of the results. (A short footnote is also provided with slightly more explanation of the technique for the interested reader.)[1] Figure 1.1 is the biplot display, on which the tribes are represented by dots, and the variables (birth and death rates, for instance) by arrows. The locations of the dots represent the similarities and differences of the tribes in relation to the variables. Thus, two close dots indicate that the corresponding tribes are similar on all variables, whereas dots that are far apart on the biplot indicate that the tribes concerned must differ considerably on at least one variable and possibly on many.

The angles formed between the arrows on the biplot reflect the correlations of the variables in the following manner. If two arrows form a small angle, they are positively correlated: that is, both variables are high for the same tribes and low for the same tribes. If, by contrast, two arrows form an obtuse angle or go in opposite directions, the variables they represent are inversely correlated: that is, tribes that have a high value of one variable will have a low value of the other. A lack of correlation between variables is represented by a right angle. It should be added that the lengths of the arrows are proportional to the variables' standard deviations, but this is not very informative in the present context in which different variables are measured in different units.

In the biplot the juxtaposition of the dots representing tribes and the arrows representing variables reflects the actual values of the original observations. To reconstruct a particular tribe's observation on a given variable (as measured from that variable's mean—the entire biplot is in terms of variation about means), drop a perpendicular line from the dot to the straight line through the arrow and measure the distance from the biplot center. Multiply this distance by the length of the arrow and add a minus sign if the perpendicular falls in the direction opposite to

TABLE 1.2
Vital Rates for Indian Tribes of Varying Types of Social Organization, 1968–1969

Service unit	Tribe	Crude death rate	Accident death rate	Infant deaths per 1,000 live births	Crude death rate minus:		Crude birth rate	Median birth order	Unemployment rate
					Accidents	Infant deaths			
1 Fort Hall	Shoshone-Bannock	19.5	4.9	55.9	14.6	16.7	49.0	3.3	56.0
2 Mescalero	Eastern Apaches	10.3	2.9	46.7	7.4	8.7	34.4	3.6	73.0
3 Jicarilla	Eastern Apaches	15.0	0.8	0	14.02	15.0	24.0	3.0	72.0
4 San Carlos	Western Apaches	12.1	2.0	44.2	10.2	10.4	40.0	3.9	47.0
5 White River	Western Apaches	7.8	1.9	50.6	5.9	6.0	35.2	4.3	70.0
6 Rosebud	Sioux	15.0	4.0	36.5	9.0	13.3	45.9	3.6	44.0
7 Pine Ridge	Sioux	12.2	2.5	24.7	9.7	11.1	44.0	4.2	63.0
8 Navajo	Navajo	6.2	1.6	45.5	4.6	4.5	33.5	4.0	56.0
9 Santa Fe	Eastern Pueblos	4.6	1.4	20.4	3.2	4.5	25.3	3.2	42.0
10 Keams	Hopis	4.3	1.1	11.4	3.2	3.9	29.7	3.1	65.0

the arrow. This multiplication reproduces the biplot approximation of the original data (as deviations from the mean). This is
useful not so much in reproducing the data matrix but in interpreting clusters of dots in the following way.

A cluster of dots represents a group of tribes with similar
observations on all variables. It is usually of interest to identify
the variables on which this cluster differs from the average or
from another cluster. This can be done on the biplot by looking
for arrows that point in the requisite direction (i.e., from the
center to the cluster or from one cluster to another). The variables represented by these arrows are the ones that account for
the differences between the clusters (K. R. Gabriel, personal
communication).

RESULTS

Table 1.1 displays the birth and death rates for 1949 to 1953
for all tribes but the Jicarilla Apaches (for which no data were
reported) and the Navajos and Hopis (for which the figures were
combined). Although the Pimas and Papagos were combined in
the original government report, I will present the data for them
here because both tribes were agricultural.

It is clear that there is a rough dichotomy between sedentary
and semisedentary agricultural tribes on the one hand and seminomadic hunting and gathering tribes on the other. The one
exception is the Pine Ridge Sioux, who have a lower death rate
than the Pima-Papagos. In general, however, the tribes that had
been hunters and gatherers in the pre- and postcontact periods
had higher average age-adjusted death rates and birth rates per
1,000 women (aged 15 to 44) in 1949–1953 than did the agricultural tribes. There is no information concerning levels of education, income, and employment for these years, so I cannot assert
that the differences observed are unrelated to involvement in the
wage economy. However, the fact that death rates in infancy do
not vary in the same way as the other rates do leads me to infer
that economic status was not consistently different between the
agriculturalists and the hunters.

The data from 1968 and 1969 are shown in table 1.2. The
figures for the Jicarilla Apaches and the Pueblos in the Santa Fe
Service Unit are only for 1968, because in 1969 they were com-

bined and cannot be distinguished. The Jicarilla population is small (about 1,300 in 1970) so the data are subject to considerable random fluctuation. The Pueblo population (about 5,800 in 1970) is larger, and the problem of random fluctuation therefore is not as significant.

Adequate data for the Paiutes, Pimas, or Papagos for this period are unavailable; therefore, these tribes are not included in table 1.2. Moreover, there are no adequate data for calculating age-specific birth and death rates. The 1970 U.S. census (U.S. Bureau of the Census 1973) gives some evidence that the Hopis and Eastern Pueblos have somewhat smaller proportions of their populations in the 0 to 24 age group than do the other tribes. However, the differences (on the order of 58 percent for Pueb-

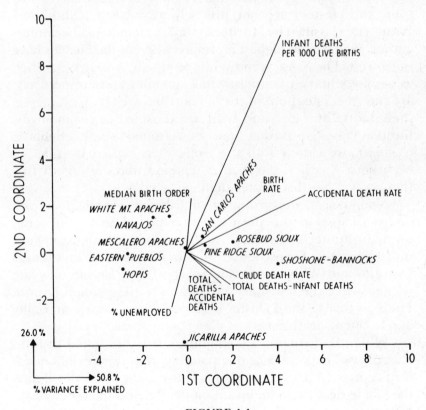

FIGURE 1.1
VITAL RATES OF AMERICAN INDIAN TRIBES, 1968—1969

los and 63 percent for the others) are not large enough to explain the differences in crude rates reported in table 1.2.

The biplot of the data in table 1.2 is shown in figure 1.1. This is a representation of the plane which explains 77 percent of the variance. At the extreme right are the Shoshone-Bannocks. To the right of the midline, the Mescalero and San Carlos Apaches and the Rosebud and Pine Ridge Sioux form a cluster. To the left of the midline the White Mountain Apaches and the Navajos form one cluster and the Eastern Pueblos and Hopis another. The Jicarilla Apaches, represented by an outlying dot, are clearly a deviant group, and I am inclined to attribute this to their small population which affords few observations and to the period of a single year for which data are available.

As hypothesized, most of the separation between tribes is accounted for by accidental deaths and crude mortality. However, the clusters are not precisely as expected; Shoshone-Bannocks, classified by Murdock (1967) as seminomadic hunter-gatherers, have the highest mortality, whereas the Pueblos have the lowest. The Navajos and White Mountain Apaches, classified as semisedentary pastoralists and agriculturalists respectively, are intermediate. Both of the Sioux tribes are above average in their mortality rates, and both are classified as seminomadic hunters. The San Carlos Apaches, classified as semisedentary, cluster more closely with the Sioux than expected, while the Mescalero Apaches, classified as seminomadic, are slightly further away from that cluster than expected.

Nonetheless, the grouping of tribes is essentially as predicted. Those in the prereservation period that were seminomadic hunter-gatherers form a loose cluster with the highest mortality rates. Semisedentary pastoralists and agriculturalists (Navajos and White Mountain Apaches) form an intermediate cluster, while the sedentary agriculturalists (Hopis and Eastern Pueblos) form a third cluster with lower than average mortality and accident death rates.

When the variables are examined, they are found to form roughly two clusters. The one pointing to the lower right quadrant represents a high correlation between the crude death rate, the crude death rate minus infant deaths, and the crude death rate minus accidental deaths. The other cluster, almost at right angles to the first, is composed of arrows representing infant mortality per 1,000 live births, the crude birth rate, the median birth order, and the accidental death rate. The proportion unemployed shows an almost perfect inverse correlation with this cluster; that is, the higher the underemployment and unemployment, the lower the infant mortality.

Infant mortality is unrelated to crude mortality or the two variables derived from it. Indeed, except for the high infant mortality of the Shoshone-Bannocks and the low infant mortality of the Pueblos and Hopis, there is no relationship between this variable and social organization. The pattern appears to be as follows: crude and accidental mortality rates are correlated, and both are ranked from high to low along the spectrum of social organization outlined immediately above. Accidental mortality is also highly correlated with crude birth rate, which also is ranked along the spectrum of social organization. The crude birth rate, however, though correlated with infant mortality, is not related to the spectrum of social organization. Presumably, infant mortality is more directly related to such variables as per capita income, housing conditions, environmental quality, and the like. Thus, fertility may be related in some complex way both to factors more directly dependent upon contemporary economic and educational conditions.

It may be objected that social organization in itself is not the underlying cause, but that other factors may be producing the relationships—for example, factors related to acculturation to the dominant society as measured by the level of education, income, and/or employment. Data on such factors are somewhat limited. I have noted above that estimates of unemployment are the only figures available for all ten reservation populations. The U.S. Census provides information on income and education for only six of the reservation populations with which we are concerned. It also provides information on all self-identified members of these tribes, whether living on or off reservations. However, some tribes are grouped so that it is not possible to provide information for each one separately. The available data are displayed in tables 1.3 and 1.4.

Information on income and education is not available for the reservation populations of Fort Hall, Mescalero, Jicarilla, or the Pueblos in the Santa Fe Service Unit because population data on the Fort Hall Shoshone-Bannocks are grouped with other re-

TABLE 1.3
INCOME AND EDUCATION OF RESERVATION POPULATIONS, 1970

Service unit	Median years of education adults > 25	Percent high school graduates, > 25 years of age	Percent below poverty line	Mean per capita income
Fort Hall	—	—	—	—
Mescalero	—	—	—	—
Jicarilla	—	—	—	—
San Carlos	8.4	13.5	63.8	687
White River	8.8	14.9	55.7	876
Rosebud	8.8	23.4	62.3	846
Pine Ridge	9.0	22.8	55.4	1,042
Navajo	4.1	17.4	64.5	776
Santa Fe	—	—	—	—
Keams Canyon	9.5	27.5	66.9	883

TABLE 1.4
INCOME AND EDUCATION OF TOTAL TRIBAL POPULATIONS
ON AND OFF RESERVATIONS, 1970

Tribe(s)	Median years of education	Percent high school graduates	Percent below poverty line	Mean per capita income
Shoshones	10.3	34.7	29.0	1,537
Apaches	8.9	23.3	46.8	1,204
Sioux	10.2	33.5	46.3	1,231
Navajos	5.3	18.8	60.2	886
Hopis	11.3	44.0	44.7	1,299
New Mexico Pueblos				
Keresan	10.4	37.1	37.4	1,201
Tanoan	10.0	33.8	46.1	1,334
Zuni	10.6	34.9	38.3	1,361

lated tribes, all Apaches are grouped together, and the New
Mexico Pueblos are divided into linguistic groups that are not
identical with the Pueblos in the Santa Fe Service Unit. Despite
these limitations, it seems evident that there are no consistent
trends in either education or income that correlate with the

accidental or crude mortality rates or with the crude birth rate. There is evidence, however, that suggests that infant mortality is inversely related to the proportion of adults with a high school education (Spearman's rho = $-.77$), whereas there is no relationship with mean income.

A clustering of tribes occurs according to vital rates and social organization, although the correlations between the vital rates are not equally high. For instance, crude death rates are not correlated with infant death rates, though they are correlated with accidental deaths. "Accidental deaths" is perhaps a misnomer, for this category also includes homicide and suicide.

The strong inverse correlation between infant mortality and employment is for me inexplicable. If employment is an indirect measure of income, and if high income is inversely related to infant mortality, as is usually the case, just the reverse correlation would have been expected. It may be that either the employment data are grossly inaccurate or the employment that does exist provides such a low level of remuneration that it has no perceptible impact on the standard of living. In addition, it may be that the income earned is spent on items having no impact on the quality of infant health. Nonetheless, the finding warrants further investigation to check its validity.

High mortality is correlated with high fertility. The fact that the correlation is highest between accidental deaths and fertility is intriguing and suggests the possibility that the same kind of impulsiveness related to accident proneness is also related to the inability or unwillingness to use contraception.

Finally, it is important to recall that not all vital rates appear to be ranked along the spectrum of social organization. Infant mortality is a conspicuous exception, and I have suggested that it is more likely to be related to socioeconomic, educational, and medical-care variables. There is only a weak inverse relationship between education and infant mortality: the higher the proportion of educated adults, the lower the infant mortality. As noted above, there is no easily understood relationship between infant mortality and unemployment or average income.

It seems reasonable, then, to suggest that fertility may be dependent upon factors related both to traditional forms of social organization—such as personality and family structure, ability to adjust to the reservation system, and the like—as well as to factors more directly related to socioeconomic status, particularly those factors that influence infant mortality. Thus, as infant mortality declines, fertility will also decline but at varying rates in part dependent upon the social organization of the particular population. Clearly, factors influencing current social and economic conditions are the most susceptible to change and, therefore, will be the most significant in reducing fertility as infant mortality is reduced. At the same time, factors related to the culture of the particular tribe in question may well influence receptivity to family planning programs even as infant mortality is reduced.

I have been concerned with reservation populations rather than with total tribal populations for which no comparable data exist. It may well be that emigration from reservations produces a consistent bias in the character of the population that remains. Pueblos, for whom ejection from the community has been a powerful mechanism of social control, may be very different from Shoshone-Bannocks in this regard. The mortality from alcoholic cirrhosis among Hopi Indians is higher than among Navajos, and most of it is found among off-reservation residents who were ejected from their home communities precisely because of their drinking behavior (Kunitz et al. 1971). For this reason I have removed from some of the calculations deaths due to so-called voluntary causes. The death rate minus accidental deaths is not highly correlated with the accident death rate, but it too tends to be ranked along the spectrum of social organization previously described. Thus, these facts confirm the notion that social organization is related to what I have perhaps inappropriately called voluntary (or accidental) causes of death, and to all other causes as well. "Preparedness," then, may be related to general susceptibility to disease as well as to what are more commonly regarded as the "social pathologies" (Levy and Kunitz 1971).

Preparedness is a tautological concept, though a useful one. Differences in mortality are a measure of preparedness for life as subordinate members of a colonial society, and I have argued that mortality differences show that preparedness differs from tribe to tribe. I have not, however, provided an independent measure of preparedness.

The mortality patterns I have described are relatively new.

Until a generation ago, epidemic diseases were the most significant causes of mortality. In the recent past, public health measures and medical services have eliminated these diseases so that others of a psychosocial nature have gained significance. While the causes of mortality may be new, the factors predisposing to greater or lesser susceptibility are rooted in ecological adaptations made centuries ago.

In this chapter I have shown that contemporary mortality patterns are the product of the way populations with different types of social organization adjust to life on reservations. In the next several chapters I will analyze changes in the Navajo economy, epidemiology, and health care practices. In the final chapter I return to the issues presented in this chapter and suggest that contemporary causes of mortality among the Navajos will be much less responsive to medical intervention than were the infectious diseases of the previous period precisely because the contemporary causes are so intimately bound up with traditional Navajo values and ways of life.

2

Economic and Demographic Change on the Navajo Reservation

THE PRERESERVATION PERIOD

NAVAJOS probably entered north-central New Mexico during the sixteenth century. As a result of pressure from other Indians, as well as from Spaniards, Mexicans, and Anglo-Americans, they moved southwest and by the first half of the 18th century, perhaps as early as 1706, they were at Canyon de Chelly (James and Lindsay 1973). A small number may have moved even farther west (D in fig. 2.1) as early as the 1620s (Kemrer 1974:127). From 1750 to 1799 the Navajos probably settled as far west as First Mesa, on what is now the Hopi Reservation (in D in fig. 2.1). By 1867 they had moved west of Third Mesa (Kemrer 1974:129–130). Brugge (1972) maintains that by the 1780s or 1790s Navajos were using land as far west as what is now Tuba City (in G in fig. 2.1).

The Navajo expansion to lower and drier areas in southwestern Colorado, southeastern Utah, and west to the Colorado and Little Colorado rivers was associated with sheepherding, which became the dominant Navajo subsistence activity by 1800 (Hester 1962:84).

Raids and warfare to capture livestock and slaves from Navajo communities were terminated in 1846 when Anglo-American

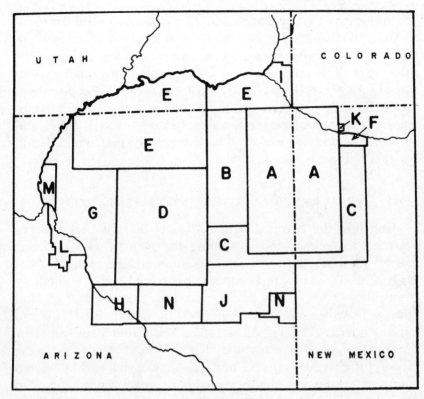

FIGURE 2.1

SUCCESSIVE ADDITIONS TO THE NAVAJO RESERVATION, 1869–1934

A: Treaty of June 1, 1868; B: Executive Order of October 29, 1878; C: Executive Order of January 6, 1880; D: Executive Order of December 16, 1882; E: Executive Order of May 17, 1884; F: Executive Order of April 24, 1886; G: Executive Order of January 8, 1900; H: Executive Order of November 14, 1901; I: Executive Order of May 15, 1905; and Act of March 1, 1933; J: Executive Orders of November 9, 1907, and January 28, 1908; K: Executive Order of December 1, 1913; L: Executive Orders of January 19, 1918, and May 23, 1930, and Act of June 14, 1934; M: Act of May 23, 1930; N: Act of June 14, 1934 (after Underhill 1963:149.)

control was introduced. When the Americans entered the scene, warfare became "exterminationist" (Kemrer 1974:135). The most devastating campaign was led by Kit Carson in 1863–64, a campaign that destroyed livestock, crops, and people, and resulted in the incarceration of 8,000 Navajos at the Bosque Redondo from 1864 to 1868.

Assuming that perhaps 2,000 Navajos were never captured, in 1864 the population was about 10,000. Hester (1962:86) estimates that in 1700 there were about 2,000 Navajos. Thus, during 160 years their numbers increased fivefold. This rapid growth apparently was due to the growing importance of sheepherding, the acquisition of agricultural techniques from the Pueblos (many of whom joined the Navajos after the revolt of 1680), and the relative isolation which protected the Navajos from raids and especially from epidemics.

THE EARLY RESERVATION PERIOD: 1868–1929

In 1868 the Navajos signed a treaty that allowed them to return to a reservation straddling the New Mexico–Arizona border (A in fig. 2.1). Since their traditional land to the east was largely occupied by Anglo-Americans, many Navajos from those areas also settled on the reservation or to the west of it on land that in 1882 became a reservation (D in fig. 2.1) for Hopis and other Indians (Kemrer 1974:136). Earlier that year Inspector C. H. Howard had estimated that 8,000 Navajos were living beyond their reservation boundaries in Arizona, and he recommended "extension of the reservation under a new agency to look after both the Hopis and the western Navajos" (Brugge 1972:17–18).

As figure 2.1 shows, large additions were made to the reservation over the next twenty years, and smaller additions continued to be made until the 1930s. Most of this land had been used prior to the nineteenth century by Navajos and other tribes, including Yavapais, Havasupais, Paiutes, and Hopis (Brugge 1972). This was particularly true in the area of Tuba City (in area G of fig. 2.1), where water and farming had existed for centuries.

After the return of the Navajos from the Bosque Redondo, sheep were provided by the government, and the flocks increased rapidly. At the same time, the Southwest entered a period of reduced rainfall, which, combined with heavy grazing, had unfortunate consequences for the range land, particularly because herds of horses also increased considerably in the 1880s and 1890s. Warnings about the problem of overgrazing came as early as 1883 from an Indian agent named Dennis Riordan (Johnston 1966a:34).

The economic condition of the Navajos was declining by 1900. Comparing data from 1890 and 1915, for instance, Johnston (1966a:36–37) calculated per capita stock valuations in dollars and found virtually no change over the twenty-five-year period. However, as the value of livestock nationwide had increased about 160 percent during those years, he estimated that the real value of Navajo holdings must have declined considerably. Efforts to improve the stock by introducing improved breeding practices started in 1900 but were unsuccessful (Kelly 1968:111–112).

Though no limits were placed on the number of livestock that could be grazed, the establishment of the reservation made the acquisition of livestock more difficult. In the prereservation years a young man could improve his status by stealing stock from non-Indians and building up his flock. After 1868 this was not possible, and social mobility was diminished (Vogt 1961). Those Navajos who were able to build up large flocks upon their return from the Bosque Redondo were fortunate. As time went on, fewer people could amass a significant number of livestock, and many turned to occasional wage labor. A source of wage labor in the 1880s was the railroad, which provided job opportunities for Navajo men (Underhill 1963:191).

The 1900 census of Hopis and of Navajos living within the Executive Order Reservation showed a deficit of Navajo males (Johansson and Preston 1977), which seemed largely due to emigration from the reservation in search of work. This emigration may have been related to polygynous marriages. Nine percent of men and 17 percent of women lived in such unions. Men with numerous livestock were able to support multiple wives, whereas those without opportunities for improving their status within the reservation system were forced to work as dependents of the well-to-do or to migrate (Levy and Kunitz 1974). The census of 1900, for example, reported an off-reservation group of 106 Navajo males and 1 female.

In addition to off-reservation employment, opportunities for mobility were created by the school system. The treaty of 1868 provided for educational opportunities which were primarily in the hands of missionary groups. The Indian Bureau assumed more direct responsibility in this century by establishing on the reservation between 1900 and 1925 nine boarding schools and two day-schools (Underhill 1963:223). In 1900, fewer than 5 percent of children from 6 to 8 were enrolled in school, but by 1930 about 40 percent were enrolled (Johnston 1966*b*:359).

On the reservation, school attendance reflected the values of the parents. In 1905 the agent in Tuba City wrote: "I am told that no child has been put in school if his people could afford to support him at home. Those who have attended schools are either orphans or the children of very poor parents. Schools are not popular with the wealthy class" (Commissioner of Indian Affairs 1905:180).

The impact of the traditional stratification system on the degree to which people took up the educational system or became wage laborers was evident in a study of several different Navajo populations in the late 1960s. The adaptation of the Navajo men to the Anglo-dominated wage work world was clearly related to the livestock holdings of their parents. At the time of interview, long-term off-reservation resident respondents came from families whose parents had owned less livestock than did the parents of reservation-resident respondents (Levy and Kunitz 1974).

The livestock economy continued to decline through the 1920s.

> Although all comparisons of the data with previous figures must be viewed with extreme caution, it is apparent at least that the population of the Navaho was increasing at a faster rate than its economic assets during the period from 1915 to 1926. Whereas Paquette estimated a total per capita value of all property held by the Navahos under his jurisdiction of $1,250 in 1915, the corresponding figure obtained in the Meriam Survey of 1926 comes to only $1,058. (Johnston 1966*a*:37–38)

The result was that fewer and fewer people could subsist by raising livestock. Therefore, when the Navajos approved an oil-drilling lease in the Four Corners area in 1921, they made it clear that they expected jobs at the drilling sites (Kelly 1968:51).

Though royalties have provided the tribe with substantial income over the years, natural resource extraction has not increased employment opportunities considerably from that time to the present.

Economic conditions have varied across the reservation. Data collected in the 1920s (table 2.1) show that the Pueblo Bonito, San Juan and Navajo reservation populations on the eastern end had higher levels of per capita income than did the populations in the Western Navajo and Leupp Reservations (Leupp is H in fig. 2.1; Western Navajo is G, M, L, and most of E). The Eastern Navajos had greater accessibility to wage work and were more involved in commercial agriculture and ranching. These differences persist to the present, and we shall see that they are related to differences in morbidity, mortality and fertility.

TABLE 2.1
ANNUAL PER CAPITA INCOME AND PROPERTY VALUES (IN DOLLARS)
NAVAJO AGENCIES, 1926

Navajo agency (reservation)	Individual and tribal property[a]	Individually owned property[b]	Tribal and individual income[c]	Individual income[d]	Earned income[e]
Western Navajo	48	47	39	32	31
Pueblo Bonito	330	330	145	142	142
Leupp	812	383	34	17	17
San Juan	842	200	127	111	85
Navajo	1,945	185	135	135	135

Source: Meriam 1928
[a]p. 442 [c]p. 449 [e]p. 455
[b]p. 445 [d]p. 452

DEMOGRAPHY, 1868–1929

The Navajo population, which increased fivefold from the eighteenth to the mid-nineteenth century, again assumed its rapid growth rate following the return to the reservation in 1868. From 1870 to 1900, the average annual rate of natural increase was somewhere between 1.5 and 2.0 percent, and for

1900 to 1930 it was between 1.75 and 2.25 percent (Johnston 1966a:152).

The Navajo population increase was greater than that of their Hopi neighbors because the densely settled and unsanitary Hopi villages caused higher mortality. Navajos lived in scattered camps where they were relatively protected from epidemic diseases such as smallpox which decimated Hopi villages on several occasions (Kunitz 1974a). Among Hopi women aged eighteen to fifty-two interviewed in the 1900 census, the average parity was higher than that of the Navajos, although at the time of the interview the average number of Hopi children alive was lower than among Navajo women of the same age. The Navajo had an average of 4.4 children ever born, with 3.6 still alive, whereas the Hopi had an average of 5.7 ever born and only 2.9 still alive. These differences were observed at the time by Jacob Breid, physician for the Hopis, who wrote in his annual report for 1905:

> At the First Mesa, population 671, there were 55 births, a rate of 8.2 percent; and 53 deaths, a rate of 7.9 percent.
>
> No statistics are available with regard to the Navaho, but I am sure that the birth rate is lower and that the mortality is also lower. Tuberculosis is common, but their general condition is better and their dwellings are far more sanitary. (Commissioner of Indian Affairs 1905:165)

Reliable fertility and mortality rates are not generally available for the Navajo population, but Morgan (1973) provided data (table 2.2) from an intensively studied border community, Ramah, New Mexico. The first point to be made about this information is that with the exception of the period from 1890 to 1904, the average annual rates of natural population increase are not very different from the probable rates calculated by Johnston for the entire tribe. The discrepancy in the early years can be attributed to the fact that Ramah was then composed primarily of young people who were establishing a new community. The second point concerning these data is that infant mortality and crude death rates began to increase in the early years of the present century. Mortality data for the entire Navajo population simply do not exist for these years, and the estimates vary considerably from one source to another, as Johnston (1966a) has shown. I believe that the pattern Morgan demonstrated for the

Ramah Navajo characterized the entire population. He attributed the increasing infant mortality and crude death rates to contact with Anglos, greater exposure to infectious diseases, and the devastating influenza pandemic of 1919. The boarding schools attended by an increasing number of children were a fertile ground for epidemics, as the reports from school superintendents indicate. A school with 100 to 200 pupils commonly experienced the death of at least one child every year. The declining livestock economy may also have caused increasing malnutrition, which would have contributed to mortality. Finally, the decline in fertility may have been due to a change in the age structure of the population as a result of increased mortality; to decreased fecundity as a result of declining nutritional status; and to conscious fertility control in the face of a declining economy. Fertility remained well above mortality, however, so the population continued to grow, though at a slower rate than in the early years of the century.

TABLE 2.2

AVERAGE ANNUAL VITAL RATES OF NAVAJO POPULATION
AT RAMAH, NEW MEXICO, 1890–1929

Year	Birth rate/ 1,000	Infant mortality/ 1,000 live births	Death rate 1,000	Rate of natural increase/1,000
1890–1894	75.2		14.1	61.1
1895–1899	68.6	60	8.4	60.2
1900–1904	61.2		8.7	52.5
1905–1909	48.3		16.1	32.2
1910–1914	38.4		15.7	22.7
1915–1919	59.4	89	27.1	32.3
1920–1924	49.9		26.6	23.3
1925–1929	41.1		25.8	15.3

Source: Morgan 1973

DEPRESSION, STOCK REDUCTION, AND WAR: 1930–1945

Despite warnings from agent Riordan and others, Navajo range land continued to be overstocked and to deteriorate. Only in the 1930s, under the New Deal, was stock reduction instituted and enforced. The reservation was divided into land management districts, and the carrying capacity of the range in each district was determined. The livestock was then reduced to the limit, with the largest herds and flocks being reduced the most. David Aberle commented, "It is reasonable to infer that the long term trajectory of per capita holdings was downward prior to reduction, that there had been a fairly marked drop in the period 1930–1933, primarily because of bad weather, and that reduction caused a further drop of about the same size" (1966:61).

Promises that more land in New Mexico would be made available to the Navajo tribe induced the tribal council to support the livestock reduction. Anglo-American interest groups defeated the attempt to fulfill these promises (Parman 1976), so that reductions in the amount of livestock were not accompanied by expansion of the land base. Other efforts were made to improve the range, however, and various public works projects provided cash income to destitute families.

The people in charge of stock reduction had to ascertain how much stock was grazed on different parts of the reservation and what other resources existed. To this end, the Soil Conservation Service carried out a Human Dependency Survey in the late 1930s, which provided the first reasonably adequate set of comparative data for the reservation as a whole (with the exception of the checkerboard area in New Mexico). The units studied were land management districts, shown in figure 2.2 (U.S. Soil Conservation Service 1939). Table 2.3 lists the values of the variables measured in the survey, and figure 2.3 is a biplot display of the variables and their relationship to one another and to the land management districts (regional differences in mortality and health care utilization are discussed in subsequent chapters and will be related to the analysis described here).

The biplot allows us to visualize the data in a useful fashion. Districts 3, 5, 7, and 17, which form a continuous strip along the western and southern portion of the reservation, were all similar in having above average sheep units per capita, the largest maximum permit sizes, and above average livestock income per capita. Districts 1, 2, and 8, which form the northwestern and northern edge of the reservation, were similar to one another and also clustered loosely with districts 4, 9, 10, 11 and 14. With the exception of district 14, these areas are all contiguous, forming

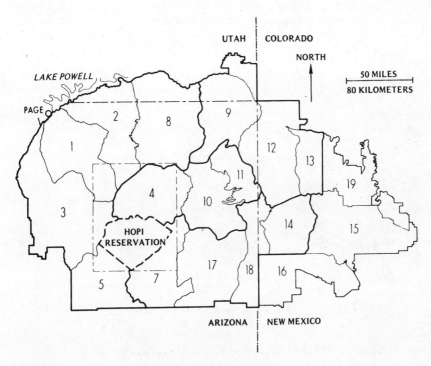

FIGURE 2.2

LAND MANAGEMENT DISTRICTS ON THE NAVAJO RESERVATION

the central area and part of the northern edge of the reservation. This entire area was characterized by large consumption groups, high noncommercial livestock income, and low involvement in the commercial and wage economy.

Districts 12, 13, and 18 were clearly different from one another and from the previous clusters. Districts 12 and 13 had above average population density and greater commercial and noncommercial agriculture. The San Juan River runs through them and some irrigation farming was practiced there. The Window Rock-Fort Defiance area was in District 18. It was the administrative center of the reservation and thus the place with greatest wage-work opportunities. Data from districts 15, 16, and 19 (the checkerboard area in New Mexico) were not uniformly available from this survey.

The population density of the eastern side of the reservation was higher than that in the west, and the people were more

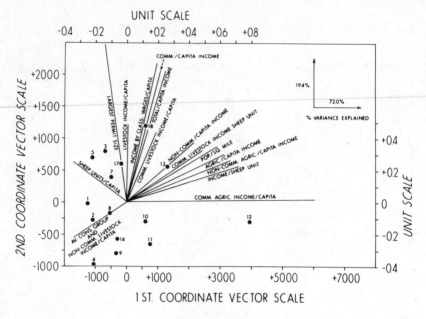

FIGURE 2.3
Biplot of Human Dependency Survey Data from the 1930s,
Navajo Reservation

involved in the wage economy and in commercial livestock and agricultural pursuits. In the west, the dominant economic activity was subsistence livestock raising, and the demographic pattern reflected this fact: fertility rates were higher (Kluckhohn and Leighton 1946) and consumption groups larger.

The most intense contact with Anglo-Americans was in the east. The western Navajos were more isolated, had less opportunity to engage in wage work and commerce, and were also less accessible to government truant officers who attempted to bring children into the boarding schools. Moreover, the population density in the east increased competition for land and thus forced families to split apart (Kimball 1965).

Cutbacks in the conservation programs (the Civilian Conservation Corps) began in 1936 and had several effects. First, wage work on the reservation decreased (Parman 1976:185–186). Second, funds were not available to maintain many schools, with the result that the proportion of school-age youngsters actually enrolled in school leveled off (Johnston 1966*b*). Finally, health

TABLE 2.3

LAND MANAGEMENT DISTRICT DATA, 1930s

LMD	A Pop./sq. mile 1936	B Avg. cons. group 1936	C Comm./capita income 1936	D Non-comm./capita income 1936	E Total/capita income 1936	F Income by class: wages/capita 1936	G Livestock income/capita 1936	H Agricult./capita income 1936	I Comm. livestock income/capita 1936	J Non-comm. livestock income/capita 1936	K Largest permit size 1930s	L Comm. agric. income/capita 1936	M Non-comm. agric. income/capita 1936	N Income/sheep unit 1936	O Comm. livest. income/sheep unit 1936	P Sheep units/capita 1936
1	.8	7.6	51.50	30.38	81.88	12.07	43.59	13.00	26.09	17.50	225	.12	12.88	1.34	.80	44.6
2	.5	7.9	65.99	42.10	108.09	28.93	36.97	27.99	22.67	14.30	161	.19	27.80	1.59	.97	31.2
3	.7	7.5	106.67	53.53	160.20	63.30	46.03	39.07	30.92	15.11	280	.65	38.42	2.36	1.58	26.7
4	1.6	8.5	35.90	34.38	70.28	5.35	34.11	21.58	21.10	13.01	72	.21	21.37	2.23	1.38	21.2
5	1.0	9.1	98.47	32.18	130.65	59.12	51.62	13.17	32.36	19.26	280	.25	12.92	2.95	1.85	25.2
7	1.3	8.0	103.82	30.59	134.41	32.04	67.32	16.87	52.65	14.67	237	.95	15.92	3.35	2.62	29.5
8	.7	7.6	83.33	49.43	132.76	55.11	37.55	30.10	17.45	20.10	154	.77	29.33	2.63	1.22	22.0
9	1.2	8.0	70.94	28.77	99.71	21.95	56.12	11.57	37.87	18.25	83	1.05	10.52	3.66	2.47	21.1
10	2.2	6.9	64.31	57.89	122.20	27.45	26.58	48.26	14.72	11.86	153	2.23	46.03	2.64	1.46	14.6
11	1.9	7.3	53.86	59.92	113.78	25.21	27.93	50.37	15.95	11.98	105	2.43	47.94	2.69	1.54	14.2
12	1.9	6.1	109.84	40.10	149.94	56.17	43.72	38.07	35.29	8.43	104	6.40	31.67	3.63	2.93	17.0
13	1.6	6.1	148.13	39.30	187.43	66.32	68.04	33.90	59.58	8.46	200	3.06	30.84	3.50	3.06	25.0
14	2.6	6.7	125.66	23.87	149.53	60.12	38.22	15.49	28.93	9.29	61	.91	14.58	2.58	1.95	19.2
17	2.1	7.0	92.62	42.88	135.50	34.71	47.45	29.61	32.79	14.66	275	1.39	28.22	3.24	2.24	20.1
18	3.0	6.2	205.69	40.40	246.09	135.25	40.63	33.75	31.94	8.69	238	2.04	31.71	2.71	2.13	20.2

programs suffered as many hospitals became outmoded and could not be repaired; a number of them were closed during World War II (Underhill 1963).

DEMOGRAPHIC CHANGE

Johnston (1966a:152) estimated that during the period between 1920 and 1950 the average annual growth rate of the Navajo population was between 2.4 and 2.8 percent. In general, Johnston's estimate for the entire tribe is congruent with Morgan's estimates of average annual rates of mortality, fertility, and natural increase for Ramah (shown in table 2.4). On the basis of studies in districts 4, 5, and 7 in the late 1930s, Kimball (1940) calculated that Navajos had a crude birth rate of 37.6 per 1,000, a crude death rate of 13.6 per 1,000, and a rate of natural increase of 24 per 1,000, also congruent with Johnston's estimates (see also Thompson 1951:34).

TABLE 2.4
AVERAGE ANNUAL VITAL RATES, RAMAH NAVAJOS

Years	Fertility/ 1,000 population	Mortality/ 1,000 population	Increase/ 1,000 population
1930–1934	45.3	20.5	24.8
1935–1939	51.2	20.2	31.0
1940–1945	51.5	23.4	28.1

Source: Morgan 1973

While the various estimates of rates of natural increase are surprisingly close, there is considerable variability between both the birth and death rates calculated by Kimball and Morgan. The most likely explanation of the differences is small sample size: about 445 at Ramah (Morgan 1973) compared with 4,000 in districts 4, 5, and 7 (Kimball 1940). The rates from Ramah are presented as five-year annual averages. The rates from districts 4, 5, and 7 are evidently for one year, most likely 1939.

If we work backwards from the rates and population sizes to calculate the actual number of births and deaths, we may do a chi-square test to determine whether the two populations (Morgan's and Kimball's study groups) are significantly different in respect of mortality and fertility. It turns out that they are not ($p>0.05$ for each). To make the point even more clearly, we may ask what population sizes we would need in order for these rates to be considered significantly different. For births, each population would have to be about 6,000; for deaths, about 10,000 (Snedecor and Cochran 1967:113, 211). Unhappily, therefore, we cannot say with any certainty whether mortality and fertility for the entire population increased, decreased, or remained essentially stable during the first four decades of this century. I believe that the Ramah data reflect a larger pattern of increasing mortality and fluctuating but generally high fertility. The continuous impressive growth of population, on which all observers agree, the continuous economic decline, and suggestive evidence (reported more fully in chapter 3) of increases in malnutrition, infant mortality, and tuberculosis all support this interpretation.

The neglect that began in the early reservation period led to increasing impoverishment as the human and livestock populations outgrew the land base and as wage work opportunities and royalties from natural resources failed to make up the difference. As elsewhere in the United States, conservation work was used both to improve the land and to employ people. From 1933 to 1936, Civilian Conservation Corps programs expanded. In 1936 they began to be cut (Parman 1976:185–186) and, concomitantly, welfare support in the form of surplus commodities began to be distributed extensively (ibid.:126–127). Shortly after Pearl Harbor, the Civilian Conservation Corps was disbanded entirely. An estimated 10,000 Navajos, however, found employment in war industries (Boyce 1974:130) and about 3,600 entered the armed services (Underhill 1963:242). The temporary substitution of a warfare for a welfare economy worked to bring more cash to the reservation from wages and soldiers' allotments. It also involved many Navajos in the larger society (Vogt 1951). If the war created something of a boom in the reservation economy, however, victory resulted in a bust that has not yet ended.

THE POSTWAR PERIOD

LATE 1940s AND 1950s

Shortly after the end of World War II, a combination of severe weather, the return of large numbers of discharged veterans and unemployed workers, and the cessation of soldiers' allotments and migrant workers' remittances brought about an economic disaster requiring emergency relief. Beyond the emergency measures that were taken, long-term planning for the rehabilitation of the tribe was initiated. The Krug Report of 1948 outlined the government's vision of the direction in which such steps should proceed and described the hoped-for results:

> In a real sense, the work with the Indians cannot be considered completed until they have been assimilated into the general population. This program for the Navajos is a long step toward assimilation. Under the squalid circumstances in which these 61,000 have been required to live and against a present background of dominant illiteracy, however, this program should be considered only as the first step toward the goal. This program should provide a satisfactory economic base on which to build the competence of the tribe. Before its completion a second, and perhaps a final step should be prepared and adopted in order that our duties to these people may be fully discharged. (Krug 1948)

The report estimated that of the approximately 61,000 Navajos, only 35,000 could be supported on the reservation at minimum subsistence, even when the resource base was developed to its maximum. That is to say, of the estimated 12,000 Navajo families, about 6,950 could be made self-sufficient on the reservation in the ways shown in table 2.5.

The remaining 5,050 families would be supported in a variety of ways, including migration to the Colorado River Reservation, and possibly further development of irrigation projects such as the Shiprock–San Juan, Animas–La Plata, and South San Juan. Even if 1,000 families moved to the Colorado River Reservation and 2,600 more could be provided for by the Shiprock–San Juan Project, there would still remain 1,450 families who would have to resettle off the reservation, according to the report's estimate (ibid.).

The recommendations of the report were intended to lead to the termination of the Navajos' special legal status and to their integration in the larger society. This was the goal of federal Indian policy throughout the late 1940s and 1950s. A large number of Navajos were supposed to become small independent farmers; others might accept relocation to cities where they were supposed to find a place in the urban labor force; and families

TABLE 2.5
PROJECTED SOURCES OF SUPPORT ON THE NAVAJO RESERVATION, 1948

	Number of families
Range improvement and soil conservation to permit maximum safe utilization of range lands	2,400
Extension of existing small irrigation projects	1,500
Further development of timber resources and enlargement of tribal sawmill	500
Coal mining and related activities	500
Development of minerals other than coal	300
Increased production and improved marketing of Navajo arts and crafts	500
General on-reservation employment (by Indian Service traders, mission schools and stations, and other nongovernmental organizations)	750
Community enterprises and industries such as canning, weaving, tourist developments, and tribal stores	500
Total	6,950

Source: Krug 1948

remaining on the land that had been the reservation were to find support from the development of natural resource extraction, small businesses, and government employment. The rapid rate of Navajo population growth (estimated at between 2.4 and 2.8 percent per year between 1920 and 1950) was not discussed in the report, but it must have been clear to many people even then that no serious consideration had been given to providing employment opportunities equal to the number of people entering the labor pool each year.

The recommendations of the Krug Report were embodied in the Navajo-Hopi Long Range Rehabilitation Act (P.L. 81-474) passed in 1950. The funds authorized by Congress for this legislation and the percentages actually allocated through 1962 are shown in table 2.6. Over 90 percent of the money authorized for schools, health facilities, roads, communications, and common service facilities (warehouses, garages, office space for district supervisors, and consolidated shops) was allocated. Between 50 and 90 percent of the money authorized for water development, irrigation projects, range improvement, resettlement on

TABLE 2.6
AMOUNTS AUTHORIZED AND ALLOCATED FROM P.L. 81-474

Purpose	Amount authorized	Percent allocated
School construction	$ 25,000,000	99.9
Health facilities	4,750,000	100.00
Roads & trails	40,000,000	95.5
Communications	250,000	100.0
Common service facilities	500,000	99.0
Subtotal	70,500,000	97.5
Agency, institutional & domestic water	2,500,000	54.2
Irrigation projects	9,000,000	73.5
Range improvement	10,000,000	70.9
Colorado River Reservation resettlement	5,750,000	59.9
Natural resource surveys	500,000	87.3
Subtotal	27,750,000	68.3
Industrial & business development	1,000,000	23.8
Off-reservation placement & relocation	3,500,000	5.5
Revolving loan fund	5,000,000	36.0
Housing & necessary facilities & equipment	820,000	3.2
Subtotal:	10,320,000	21.8
Total:	108,570,000	82.8

Source: TNY 1961:5

the Colorado River Reservation, and natural resource surveys was allocated. Less than 50 percent of the money authorized for industrial and business development, off-reservation placement, the revolving loan fund, and housing was allocated.

In terms of both absolute amounts authorized and percentages actually allocated, service facilities and roads received most attention; range conservation, irrigation, business and industrial development, and relocation received considerably less. This pattern reflects the direction largely taken by the reservation economy right up to the present. What was to be developed was not a viable local economy but one dependent upon welfare and employment in the service sector.

The economic picture remained bleak throughout the 1950s. Between 1951 and 1960 the irrigation projects led to the development of 124 new farms benefiting 620 individuals (TNY 1961:125). A few small industries were attracted to the reservation and to border towns, but none employed as many as 50 Navajos at a time during the decade and one—an electronics firm—closed during the business recession of 1956–57 (TNY 1961:192). Between 1945 and 1951, 116 Navajos moved to the Colorado River Reservation; none moved there between 1952 and 1960. Between 1950 and 1960, 72 Navajos withdrew, leaving 44 still on the Colorado River Reservation at the end of 1960.

During the decade of the 1950s, 3,273 Navajos were relocated to urban areas under the auspices of the BIA and the Tribe. About 35 percent returned to the reservation during the follow-up period (usually about twelve months). It is not known how many migrated without support of the Tribe and the BIA, nor how successful they were in adjusting to the communities to which they moved. A number of studies of off-reservation Navajos have been reviewed by Henderson and Levy (1975). The general impression from the most comprehensive and sophisticated of these (of migrants to Denver) is that return rates continued to be high during the 1960s and that the Navajo migrants' economic position remained marginal.

The continued population growth during the 1950s and early 1960s (estimated at between 2.4 and 3.3 percent per year), the failure to significantly expand the land base, and the continuing decline in the quality of range land led to a further decline in the livestock economy. In 1915, 24.2 percent of the population of the Southern Navajo (Fort Defiance) Agency had owned no livestock. By 1958 the percentage reservationwide was 53.9 (TNY 1961:212).[1] At the same time as the livestock economy declined and a viable local wage economy failed to materialize, a provision in the Long Range Rehabilitation Act allowed the federal government to reimburse the states for their support of categorical welfare programs for Navajos and Hopis (aid to dependent children, the needy blind, and the aged). In addition, the growth of schools and the transfer of health care to the Division of Indian Health of the U.S. Public Health Service meant that the social service sector of the economy would continue to expand. Indeed, by the mid-1950s over 90 percent of Navajos aged six to eighteen were enrolled in school (Johnston

1966*b*:359). Thus, not only did welfare support become increasingly available, but what jobs there were for Indians tended to be in the service sector of the local economy.

By 1960 distribution of sources of individual Navajo income were estimated as follows: earned cash income, 68 percent; unearned cash income, 11.8 percent; and unearned noncash income, 19.3 percent. Estimated per capita cash income was $521, and total per capita (including noncash) income about $645. This was about 30 percent of per capita income in McKinley County, New Mexico and about 25 percent of the per capita income of the general U.S. population (TNY 1961:228–229). These estimates for the entire reservation are confirmed by a detailed study of one isolated community from the same period. In 1961–62 at Navajo Mountain in the northwestern portion of the reservation, wage income was estimated at 26.6 percent of the total, and unearned cash and noncash income together totaled about 32.2 percent (Shepardson and Hammond 1964). So-called traditional income (livestock and agriculture) accounted for about 39 percent of the total. Thus, it would appear that unearned income accounted for about 30 percent of the total.

Equally significant is that, excluding unearned income and considering only earned cash income, 37.3 percent came from service institutions such as the BIA, the PHS, the public school system, and the Tribe (excluding the Forest Products Industry) (TNY 1961:228). In other words, 25.7 percent of all Navajo income came from employment in the service sector, and about 30 percent came from unearned benefits provided by the service sector.

1960S TO THE PRESENT

The tumultuous decade of the 1960s did not leave the Navajos unaffected. In response to the civil rights movement and urban disorders, the federal government declared a War on Poverty. Concurrently, the undeclared war in Viet Nam led to a growth in war-related industries such as electronics. Finally, the energy crisis and increasing dependence on foreign sources of fuel led to a growing interest in the use of natural resources on the Navajo Reservation, including coal, oil, and uranium.

The War on Poverty on Indian reservations was administered by the Office of Economic Opportunity, called the Office of Navajo Economic Opportunity (ONEO) on the Navajo Reservation. For the most part, the programs of ONEO were a supplement to the social service programs of the BIA and the PHS. As in other poverty areas such as urban and rural ghettos, ONEO programs both created new careers in human services and provided direct services. These programs differed from those of the established agencies in being initiated by local groups.

A look at the budgets of the major agencies on the reservation in the early 1970s suggests the magnitude of these service-related expenditures. In 1972 the BIA budget for the Navajo Area was 108.9 million dollars, of which 70.2 percent was spent for education and welfare. The Indian Health Service budget for the Area was 26 million dollars, all of which was for health-related services. The ONEO budget (in 1971) was 7.9 million dollars, most of which again was spent on services such as prevocational training (34 percent), Project Headstart (28.2 percent), alcoholism treatment programs (5 percent), emergency food and medicine (4.4 percent), and similar smaller programs. In addition, numerous new job categories were created: social service aide, mental health worker, alcoholism worker, legal aide, veterinary aide, teacher aide, community health representative, physicians' assistants, and so on. Some were sponsored by the established agencies, many by ONEO. Finally, the Navajo tribal budget was 23.8 million dollars, of which 25.8 percent was spent on human development (health and welfare, veterans' affairs, social security, etc.) and another 7 percent on education. Thus, virtually all the federal money spent on the reservation and a significant proportion of the tribal budget were devoted to human and social services and to the employment of Navajos in these programs (Ruffing 1974; Kunitz 1977).

A number of manpower surveys show the impact of these spending patterns. A study in 1967 found that of 8,300 wage or salaried Navajo workers, 65.8 percent were employed in the service or government sector, excluding tribal employees in enterprises such as forest products (Navajo Tribe 1968:25f.). A second survey in 1969 by the Arizona State Employment Service showed that 68.3 percent of those with nontraditional employment worked for the federal (32.9 percent), state and local (11.9 percent), or tribal (23.5 percent) governments. Again tribal employees in productive enterprises are not included, and the figures represent essentially service workers (Reno 1970:9).

More recent data published by the Navajo Tribe (1974:23) show that 66 percent of employed Navajos are in public services; this contrasts with the 53.8 percent of non-Navajo reservation residents in public services. The non-Navajo percentage is small primarily because about 73 percent of construction workers on the reservation were non-Navajos, largely because of union membership requirements on construction jobs and the low union participation and skill levels of reservation Navajos.

Even with a greater participation in unions, however, the situation would not have been changed radically (Robbins 1975). Of the 20,140 Navajo and non-Navajo individuals in wage, salaried, or self-employed positions on the reservation, 12,613 (62.6 percent) were in public services (Navajo Tribe 1974:23). Thus even if all available jobs were held by Navajos, the wage economy would still have been based primarily on services (Kunitz 1977). As Glenn (1976:44) has noted, "At the present time, then, the largest single 'industry' in the Navajo Nation is education, and the second largest industry is public administration."

These data pertain only to employed Navajos. When the entire labor force is considered, unemployment and under-employment rates combined are between 50 and 60 percent. Thus, despite the additional federal money allocated for economic development throughout the 1960s, unemployment remained high and the employment that did exist was almost entirely within the service sector. In general, when jobs are created, they tend to be in labor-intensive rather than in capital-intensive areas. Labor intensiveness is characteristic of the service sector, which may be one reason for its expansion, but it is also true of other sectors. Writing of Indian reservations, Sorkin (1971:89) has noted:

> Because reservation labor costs are relatively low, most of the industries that have located there are labor-intensive, highly competitive ones, manufacturing products such as furniture, garments, fishhooks and fishnets, wooden items, costume jewelry, baskets, Indian artifacts, and electrical components.

This pattern appeared to change slightly during the Viet Nam war which saw the federally subsidized movement of electrical component plants to reservations. To quote Sorkin (1971:80):

> After 1963 there was an acceleration in reservation industrial development, which generally paralleled the rapid economic growth of the nation. Defense spending, bolstered by the needs of the Viet Nam war, stimulated the establishment of approximately a dozen electronic plants making circuits and transistors partly for military purposes.

Several of these new plants were built on or near the Navajo reservation: one in Page, Arizona, another at Fort Defiance, and a third in Shiprock, New Mexico. By the mid-1970s, only the Fort Defiance plant was still operating. As noted earlier, however, even when all three plants were in operation in the 1960s, they did not employ enough people to lower unemployment significantly or to alter the composition of the employed labor force.

Indian involvement in the service sector was further increased in 1975 when the Indian Self-Determination and Education Assistance Act (P.L. 93-638) was passed. Title I, the Indian Self-Determination Act, created mechanisms whereby tribes could, if they wished, contract with the Secretaries of Interior and Health, Education, and Welfare to develop new services or to assume control over services previously provided by the federal government. For the most part these were educational or health programs; management of natural resources remained more firmly under the control of the Department of the Interior.

P.L. 93-638 was accepted by conservatives who favored reducing federal government subsidies of reservation social services and physical maintenance and who supported assimilation as a means to that end. It was also accepted by many Indians as a means of developing greater self-government (Guillemin 1980). The paradoxical results have been an intensification of "tribal competition for federal support" and a narrowing of "political concerns to the managerial problems of social service programs. Rather than assisting tribes by expanding options of self-reliance, self-determination policy has deepened tribal dependence on central government funding and possessions. At the same time, the power of the BIA to represent tribal interests has declined, producing an overflow of tribal-specific conflicts in the courts" (Guillemin 1980:29). In addition, the growing concern with managerial problems of social service agencies has produced cadres of tribal grantsmen with personal and bureaucratic ties to a variety of federal agencies on which continuing support depends (Levy and Kunitz 1981).

A number of tribal leaders felt this program would result in self-termination rather than self-determination, and some tribes have therefore elected not to develop their own programs on contract to the government. They feared, for instance, that contracts might be so strictly audited that were mistakes found, the contract might be ended, leaving the tribe worse off than before. Or that contracts might not allow for increasing costs and hence the amount available would decline, creating pressure on the tribe to make up the difference out of its own revenues—especially since overhead expenses for the tribes are higher than for federal agencies and the law stipulates that tribally provided services must be at least as complete as those previously available.

A year after the passage of P.L. 93-638, P.L. 94-437, the Indian Health Care Improvement Act, was enacted. The purpose of this act was not only to build new facilities but to help create new and needed services and to attract more Indians into health-related occupations. In combination, the two acts have increased hiring of Indians in health and education programs, encouraged Indian students to pursue careers in these fields, and established tribal bureaucracies to manage government contracts.

An evaluation of the full impact of these pieces of legislation is beyond my purpose here. Without a doubt, however, they have worked to reinforce the service-oriented structure of the reservation economy. What is unfortunate is not that Indians have been able to get jobs in health, education, and welfare programs but rather that service programs have not been balanced by equal growth in more productive sectors of the economy.

The general failure of the Navajo economy even to keep pace with that of the nation overall is reflected in the comparative income figures displayed in tables 2.7 and 2.8. Between 1969 and 1974, Navajo per capita income decreased relative to national per capita income. Median family income did not change much as a percentage of the national figures, however, indicating in part that what money is available to the generally large Navajo

TABLE 2.7
NAVAJO AND U.S. INCOME IN CURRENT DOLLARS

Mean per capita income	1959	1969	1974
Navajo	$ 521	$ 753	$ 834
U.S.	$1,905	$3,130	$ 4,400
Navajo as percent of U.S.	27.3	24.1	19.0
Median family income			
Navajo	$1,548	$3,535	$ 3,601
U.S.	$5,417	$9,433	$12,800
Navajo as percent of U.S.	28.6	37.5	28.1

Source: Wistisen et al. 1975

families must be spread more thinly than is true for families nationwide. In terms of constant dollars, Navajo income is not only lower than that of the general U.S. population, but the gap between them is widening, and the Navajos were worse off in 1974 than they were in 1969 (table 2.8).

While the data provided here pertain to the entire reservation population, it is clear that there are intrareservation differences that should be kept in mind. Recall that in the 1930s virtually the entire population, except in districts 12, 13, and 18, was dependent upon livestock. Though differences did exist among the other land management districts, they tended to be fairly similar along the parameters measured. When we examine available economic data for 1974 (table 2.9), however, using the same graphic technique, we notice much less clustering of the

TABLE 2.8
NAVAJO AND U.S. INCOME IN 1967 DOLLARS

Mean per capita income	1959	1969	1974
Navajo	$ 597	$ 686	$ 567
U.S.	$2,182	$2,831	$2,991
Median family income			
Navajo	$1,773	$3,219	$2,448
U.S.	$6,205	$8,591	$8,702

Source: Wistisen et al. 1975

land management districts along the measured parameters. The variables used for 1974 are not the same as in those used for the 1930s, reflecting a decline in the significance of livestock and agriculture and an increase in the significance of wage work and welfare (the selection and source of variables are discussed in appendix I). Suffice it to say here that along with the measure of distance from hospitals (see table 2.9), the parameters are the independent variables used in the multiple regression analyses described in subsequent chapters; various measures of mortality and hospital utilization form the dependent variables.

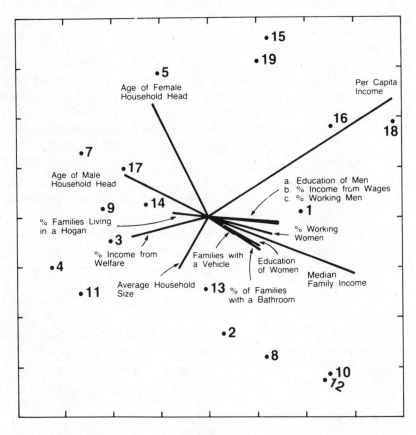

FIGURE 2.4

BIPLOT DISPLAY OF 1974 ECONOMIC VARIABLES
BY LAND MANAGEMENT DISTRICT, 1974

Looking at the biplot, notice that there are positive correlations between the vectors representing per capita and median income, male and female educational levels, degree of dependence upon wage work, and the availability of motor vehicles and indoor toilets (the last highly correlated with the presence of other domestic conveniences; see appendix I). In general, districts to the right of the midline have populations with above average incomes and education, as well as with domestic conveniences and motor vehicles. To the left of the midline are populations above average in age, household size, dependence upon welfare, and the degree to which they live in hogans rather than in nontraditional dwellings.

For the most part, the western districts house the older populations heavily dependent on welfare, whereas the eastern districts comprise the younger, better educated, wage working populations. There are exceptions, however. Northwestern districts 1, 2, and 8 are more like eastern than other western districts, presumably because of increasing wage work opportunities in Page, Kayenta, and on Black Mesa. And districts 9, 11, and 17 are more like western than other eastern districts. Nonetheless, it is accurate to say that, with some exceptions, those districts that forty years ago had populations dependent upon subsistence livestock raising now have populations dependent upon welfare; where commercial and wage work activities were observed forty years ago, they still exist.

ECONOMIC CHANGE AND SOCIAL ORGANIZATION

I have shown so far that (1) the Navajo economy has come to depend increasingly upon unearned income and wage work, and livestock has assumed less significance in the support of more people; (2) the population has grown at a rapid rate throughout the reservation period; and (3) economic development has occurred only fitfully and in a boom-bust pattern in response to changes in the national economy.

A number of observers of the Navajos and other Indian populations (Aberle 1963, 1969, 1981; Jorgensen 1971; Robbins 1975; Lamphere 1979) have argued that this pattern of economic nondevelopment has encouraged the persistence of kin networks, which provide mutual support to members and serve

TABLE 2.9
ECONOMIC DATA, 1974

LMD	Miles to nearest		Percent of income from		Education of household head		Percent living in Hogan	Percent with bathroom	Average household size	Percent working > 50 weeks/year		Percent with Vehicle	Income median per		Age of household head	
	Hospital	Surgery	Wages	Welfare	Male	Female				Male	Female		Family	Capita	Male	Female
1	44.5	55.6	73.7	21.1	9.2	9.6	24.4	28.9	6.3	42.1	9.5	56.6	3,714	954	43.5	40.9
2	77.1	89.6	64.7	31.6	8.2	9.1	17.1	14.3	6.2	50.0	9.1	82.4	3,585	735	45.3	38.9
3	27.2	27.2	42.1	22.6	7.2	6.4	23.6	25.0	8.7	15.0	3.6	55.6	3,107	635	45.9	43.6
4	79.2	121.2	48.2	40.7	7.4	7.6	35.7	1.2	6.5	24.1	8.3	47.1	2,523	554	47.2	41.7
5	47.0	94.3	57.0	10.5	6.8	6.9	12.1	6.1	6.1	12.0	12.1	53.1	3,283	791	48.8	45.8
7	40.2	101.3	51.0	28.8	7.7	7.3	20.3	11.7	6.1	19.6	3.4	50.0	2,616	632	47.1	45.2
8	36.9	110.7	72.5	13.9	8.5	9.0	23.4	26.2	7.5	56.6	12.5	58.5	3,876	703	41.8	40.4
9	59.5	59.5	47.5	27.8	7.8	8.8	15.9	7.9	8.0	32.1	1.7	68.9	2,303	677	46.9	42.6
10	46.6	61.4	77.5	12.0	9.8	11.0	7.2	46.4	7.0	46.6	16.5	69.8	4,209	786	43.9	39.1
11	60.6	69.4	46.1	23.1	6.9	7.2	17.1	20.0	7.6	22.6	2.9	57.1	3,239	487	47.1	43.7
12	28.9	28.9	71.4	7.5	8.9	9.1	4.3	37.4	7.4	41.7	26.5	71.8	4,453	740	42.9	40.2
13	40.9	40.9	70.9	11.4	8.3	8.4	11.8	32.4	6.4	38.5	11.8	61.8	3,470	640	45.3	42.2
14	41.3	41.3	49.1	9.7	8.8	9.0	5.1	20.0	6.7	42.1	11.7	58.3	3,150	593	48.5	45.0
15	33.2	84.6	75.0	14.1	9.0	7.9	21.4	17.9	4.1	53.3	10.3	62.1	2,830	1,004	44.8	43.9
16	18.6	24.5	69.1	15.2	8.7	8.6	17.5	21.2	5.0	58.3	15.8	67.3	4,098	1,003	44.6	43.3
17	22.1	54.0	57.1	19.5	8.2	7.2	21.5	15.2	6.1	50.0	5.1	44.3	3,028	600	45.6	46.4
18	20.6	20.6	69.5	7.8	10.3	9.5	14.9	34.1	5.3	48.1	19.3	54.1	4,752	1,074	44.6	43.8
19	82.2	103.2	65.2	11.3	7.9	8.3	7.0	18.6	4.8	44.1	9.3	74.4	3,024	949	44.9	44.8
Unweighted Mean 44.8	66.0		61.5	18.3	8.3	8.4	16.7	21.4	6.4	38.8	10.5	60.7	3,403	753	45.5	42.8
Symbol NEARH	NEARS		WAGE	WELF	EDM	EDF	HOGAN	BATH	HSIZE	WORKM	WORKF	VEHIC	MED-INC	PER-CAP	AMHH	AFHH

Source: Wistisen et al. 1975

to redistribute income from multiple and unstable sources. That these networks and extended families persist even in the absence of significant numbers of livestock suggests that they are adaptive to the current economic situation.

Aberle, for instance, has written that

> The effects of all these factors promoting under-development in the Navajo country are, at the local level, a particular style of economic and social life—often criticized by Anglos as evidence of backwardness, or praised by some as "the Navajo way." It has some roots in custom, but it has its present causes in current economic conditions and represents an adjustment to them. . . .
>
> The key items that promote the Navajo style are—(1) shortages of material equipment, stemming from a shortage of cash; (2) simple logistic problems in running the household and the subsistence economy, resulting from a need for some wage labor and from the difficulties involved in herding, getting water, and hauling fuel; and (3) fluctuating income. (Aberle 1969: 243–245)

As he explains, the shortage of equipment, such as a pickup truck, requires that a cluster of families pool their resources to pay for its purchase and maintenance. The need to haul firewood and water and to herd sheep may necessitate the pooling of labor, for which a "cluster of families (the extended family)" is again useful. The fluctuations in income, which result from the vagaries of weather and disease, from variations in the price of wool, mohair, sheep, and cattle, from periodic reevaluation of eligibility for welfare support, and from the unstable nature of employment, all encourage the "Navajo style."

> Not only is there continual gift giving and borrowing within the extended family to cope with these variations, but there is a wide circle of kin who depend on each other, who ask for help when they need it and give help when they can. This style of economic life we may call reciprocity—the Navajos call it "helping out" when they speak of it in English—and the ethic that accompanies it is generosity.
>
> Thus in a typical extended family—parents, some of their children (usually daughters) and their mates, and their children's children—multiple economic dependencies are the rule: livestock,

farming, weaving, part-time off-reservation work, and welfare are frequently found as income and subsistence sources in the same unit. No one of these can be relinquished—that is, efficient specialization is impossible—because none is certain and none is sufficient. (Aberle 1969:245)

It has been hypothesized that the availability of steady jobs encourages the development of independent nuclear households whereas unstable employment encourages dependence upon a variety of sources of income and continuing reciprocity among kin for the redistribution of income. Families interviewed by members of the Lake Powell Research Project in districts 1, 3, 4, and 8 varied in their degrees of independence from kin, but even those skilled workers with a history of relatively stable employment who would have been expected to be the most autonomous, as a result of their migratory patterns following construction jobs, still acknowledged continuing economic obligations to a variety of kin. Virtually all provided some form of support to parents, in-laws, and/or siblings, and many maintained small numbers of livestock at home as well. This behavior may be seen as a hedge against the unemployment that many Indians seem to feel is inevitable in the unstable economy in which they live (Levy 1980). It is still true, however, that those individuals least embedded in kinship networks seem to be the ones with the history of fullest employment, whereas those individuals with a less favorable employment history and with income from multiple sources tend for the most part to live in extended families of a variety of types. I infer that stability of income is the cause of (or makes possible) the gradual severing of kinship obligations.

As Callaway has noted,

All those household types which are in a clear majority in Anglo Society—single individual, conjugal pair and independent nuclear households—are based upon adequate and steady incomes. These same household types are characterized by high employment among the Navajo. Those household types which comprised 49 percent of our sample and represented a pooling of assorted kin have nearly double the unemployment rate of the other more independent household types. (Callaway, in press)

DEMOGRAPHIC CHANGES IN THE POSTWAR YEARS

FERTILITY RATES

Fertility rates from Ramah, New Mexico (table 2.10) suggest a slow decline over the twenty years 1945 to 1964. The average annual rate calculated for the Many Farms (district 10) population in the late 1950s was about 48.7 per 1,000 (McDermott et al. 1960). For the entire tribe the reporting of births was inadequate until at least the mid-1950s (Johnston 1966a; Hadley 1955). Thus the reasonably close agreement between the Many Farms and Ramah data is comforting and supports the conclusion that at least into the early 1960s crude fertility for the entire tribe was unlikely to have been less than 40 per 1,000.

TABLE 2.10
AVERAGE ANNUAL VITAL RATES OF RAMAH NAVAJOS, 1945–1964

Year	Average annual birth rate	Average annual death rate	Average annual rate of natural increase
1945–1949	45.0	15.3	29.7
1950–1954	41.9	12.0	29.9
1955–1959	41.1	6.3	34.8
1960–1964	40.7	6.5	34.2

Source: Morgan 1973

Since the early 1960s reporting has improved considerably as 95 percent or more of births occur in hospitals. Unpublished reports furnished by the Indian Health Service as well as my own studies of hospital records suggest that the number of births to Navajo women in the years 1971 to 1974 was between 4,000 and 4,200 per year. Assuming a resident population of 130,000 in 1974 (Faich 1977), the crude birth rate would have been approximately 31 or 32 per 1,000 in that year. Thus, while the data are far from adequate, it appears safe to say that fertility rates have declined gradually over the past thirty years.

It is possible to draw age-specific fertility rate curves and to categorize them into three types (United Nations 1965; DeJong 1972). The broad peak type is said to be characteristic of developing nations in which birth rates in the 20–24 and 25–29 age groups differ very little, are higher than the rates in groups above and below those ages, and decline in the older age groups as a result of menopause. The early peak type shows highest fertility rates in the 20–24 age group, and the late peak type shows highest rates in the 25–29 age group. The early and late peak curves both show rapid declines in fertility at all ages above 30 and are said to be characteristic of developed nations. Generally, peak fertility occurs in the twenties; this is said to be the case in virtually all populations; but continuing high fertility of women into the thirties and forties is characteristic of developing nations.

Not only are there differences over time but there are regional differences at present on the Navajo reservation in both crude and age-specific fertility rates. Figure 2.5 displays age-

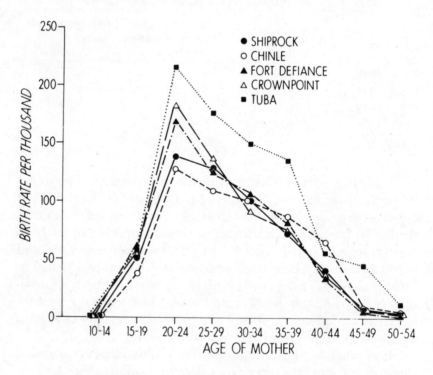

FIGURE 2.5

NAVAJO AGE-SPECIFIC BIRTH RATES BY SUB-AGENCY; FISCAL YEAR
1971–1972 AVERAGED

specific birth rate curves for Navajo women residing in different parts of the reservation in the early 1970s. Figure 2.6 is a map of the geographic regions (agencies) in which the women live. The population estimates on which the rates are based come from the BIA's population register, which has been shown to overestimate the population size. Thus, the rates reported are probably lower than the actual rates, but what is of concern here are the regional differences in the configurations of the curves, which I believe are valid.

It is clear that the farther west the population is located, the broader the curve and the higher the peak in the 20−24 age group (Kunitz 1974*b*). This indicates not only that fertility is higher in the economically less developed areas but that the differences are accounted for both by continued childbearing of older women and by higher fertility of younger women.

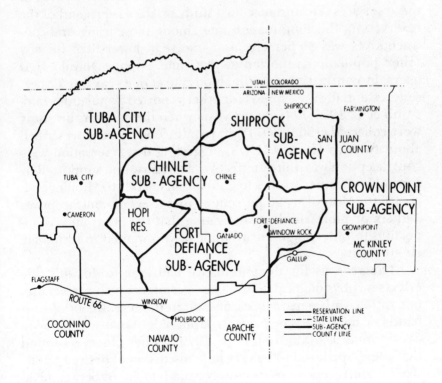

FIGURE 2.6

MAP OF NAVAJO RESERVATION SUB-AGENCIES

There is also some evidence that throughout the 1970s the rate of births to teenagers on the reservation increased, in contrast to the decline in age-specific birth rates observed in the U.S. population as a whole. Births to older women, however, continued to decline slowly during the 1970s (Temkin-Greener et al. 1981).

CONTRACEPTIVE USE

At least until recently Navajos had not used contraception frequently or effectively. Though various herbs and mechanical means to prevent or terminate pregnancies were known, these were resorted to traditionally only when the mother's health was in danger; otherwise pregnancies were carried to term (Bailey 1950). When family planning programs were first introduced in the 1960s, acceptance was hardly overwhelming and effectiveness of use was low among those who did avail themselves of these services. For instance, in a study on the eastern end of the reservation, the continuation rate among those using oral contraceptives was 35 percent after one year, lower than for any other population reported at that time. Among Navajo IUD users, by contrast, the continuation rate at one year was 72 percent, essentially the same as for other reported populations (Slocumb et al. 1975:724). In the years when the data for this study were collected (1963–1971), oral contraceptives were prescribed about twice as often as IUD's, suggesting that reservation-wide contraception was quite ineffective, an observation supported by a number of other studies (e.g., Wallach et al. 1967; Bollinger et al. 1970). Moreover, 20 percent of first users of contraceptives had six or more children, indicating that the program was appealing to older, high parity women who wanted to terminate childbearing.

The reasons for discontinuance had little to do with side effects or physiological failure (e.g., pregnancy with correct use) but rather with personal reasons, often the resentment of husbands or boyfriends or pressure from older family members to discontinue use (Slocumb et al. 1979). Other observers found that there appeared to be very little discussion of desired family size or contraceptive use within Navajo families or between Navajo patients and health care providers (Doran 1972; Khattab 1974).

Khattab (1974) suggested that the reason Navajo fertility remained high and contraceptives were not used was because in the course of the reservation period available roles for women had diminished so that their only creative outlet was childbearing. Her study was done in Ramah, the same community for which Morgan calculated the mortality and fertility patterns presented previously. Based upon those data, it is hard to claim that fertility rates did in fact increase over the reservation period, as would have been expected if Khattab's hypothesis were correct.

My alternative hypothesis is that if the culture of the kin group was compatible with that of the professional providers of care, utilization would be high, and if they were at variance, utilization would be low. In my study I conjectured that the family networks would strongly influence rates of utilization. Navajo values have generally been pronatalist, so I expected that women would be discouraged by their kin from using contraception but would be free to use it if they had enough children to wish to terminate childbearing and were relatively free of kin influence.

The results of the study—done in districts 1 and 3 where age-specific birth rates are high—supported the hypothesis but only for high parity, older, and relatively poorly educated women. In this group, the more dependent upon kin the women were, the less likely they were to use contraception (Kunitz and Tsianco 1981). Sampling biases do not allow inferences to be made about younger, low parity, well educated women. A study of utilization rates of bilateral tubal ligations and therapeutic abortions provide complementary data, however (Temkin-Greener et al. 1981).

In the years 1972 to 1978 the rate of therapeutic abortions per 1,000 deliveries increased from 33.8 to 76.5, with the greatest change observed among women below the age of 35. There was essentially no change in the rate for older women. During the same years, by contrast, tubal ligations increased from 41.3 to 46.7 per 1,000 deliveries, but it was highest in the group 35 and above (123.5 to 155.4 per 1,000). Moreover, the proportion of interval procedures (those done at a time other than immediately after delivery or abortion) increased from 15.1 to 30.7 percent, indicating that it was increasingly becoming an elective procedure planned well in advance. Multiple regression analyses of the rates of the two procedures indicate that they are highest in areas characterized by involvement in wage work where nuclear family organization is most prevalent.

The results of these studies point to several conclusions. First, the use of therapeutic abortions, tubal ligations, and contraception is low among young women generally. Second, surgical procedures are used most frequently in populations where wage work is most common and where family organization tends to be nuclear rather than extended, indicating that fertility norms are changing among the most acculturated segment of the population. Third, fertility is dropping among older women, as they increasingly use sterilizing procedures to terminate childbearing. And fourth, the persistence of extended forms of family organization as an adaptation to the harsh economic situation on the reservation has had the paradoxical effect of retarding the use of contraception among older, high parity women, the group in which fertility rates generally decline first in populations in which birth rates are beginning to drop. I suspect that extended family organization also discourages contraceptive use by young women as well. The evidence, though at the ecological level of analysis, supports this position, for rates of abortions and tubal ligations are highest in areas where family organization tends to be nuclear rather than extended.

MORTALITY PATTERNS

Average annual crude mortality rates of Ramah Navajos declined rapidly between 1945 and 1964 (table 2.10), a decline which, combined with only slowly declining fertility, resulted in a spurt in the population growth rate. The Ramah mortality figures are not very different from those calculated by Johnston (1966a:174) for the entire tribe (table 2.11). Data from the late 1960s and mid-1970s confirm the continuous decline in mortality. Table 2.12 displays estimated crude mortality rates of populations in the various Indian Health Service catchment areas. Finally, using more recent data, crude mortality in 1974 has been estimated at 6 to 7 per 1,000 (Kaltenbach 1976). With fertility at 30 to 32 per 1,000 in those years, the rate of natural increase was approximately 23 to 26 per 1,000.

Two final points must be made. First, it will be recalled that

TABLE 2.11
ESTIMATED NAVAJO CRUDE MORTALITY RATES

Year	Rate	Males ± 2 standard deviations	Rate	Females ± 2 standard deviations
1945	11.1	10.4 – 11.8	10.5	9.8 – 11.2
1950 a	11.5	11.0 – 12.0	9.9	9.4 – 10.4
b	10.6	10.1 – 11.1	9.2	8.7 – 9.2
1955	8.5	8.1 – 8.9	6.7	6.3 – 7.1

Source: Johnston 1966a:174

fertility rates have tended to be higher in the western regions of the reservation than in the east. Mortality rates, however, have not differed widely from one place to another (table 2.12). As a result, rates of natural increase have been higher in the west than in the east and, as indicated in considerable detail elsewhere, this appears to be related to higher rates of emigration from the western than from the eastern areas (Kunitz 1976a).

Indeed, Johnston (1966a:130) has shown that between 1935 and 1957, population grew most rapidly in the eastern districts. That trend appears to be continuing as young people migrate to sources of wage work both off the reservation and in eastern areas of the reservation itself. Callaway et al. (1976:21) observed that in wage work communities the population is generally younger than in more isolated communities, indicating that the same process is taking place among Navajos as among many

TABLE 2.12
NAVAJO MORTALITY RATES PER 1,000 POPULATION, 1968–1969

Service unit	Crude mortality rate
Chinle	6.9
Crownpoint	7.2
Fort Defiance	7.0
Gallup	5.8
Kayenta	7.0
Shiprock	5.6
Tuba City	8.2
Winslow	5.1

Source: Kunitz 1976a:25

other rural populations in this country: a residual population of the elderly remains as young people leave for employment elsewhere. I shall return to problems of the elderly in chapter 5.

Second, the course of Navajo mortality over the past century has been different from that of whites and nonwhites in the larger society. Among Navajos there is evidence that mortality increased from perhaps 14 to 15 per 1,000 in the 1890s to 25 to 27 per 1,000 in the late 1910s and 1920s, and then declined first gradually in the 1930s and then rapidly in the 1940s and 1950s. Crude and age-adjusted mortality for whites and nonwhites (the large majority of whom are blacks) in the United States declined steadily from 1900 through 1970, with age-adjusted rates for nonwhites remaining above those for whites each year (table 2.13). At present, mortality of Navajos, all nonwhites, and whites are very similar, though, as the next chapter will indicate, the pattern of causes differs.

TABLE 2.13
CRUDE AND AGE-ADJUSTED MORTALITY RATES OF WHITES AND NONWHITES
IN THE UNITED STATES, 1900–1970

	Age-adjusted rate/1,000		Crude rate/1,000	
Year	Whites	Nonwhites	Whites	Nonwhites
1900	17.6	27.8	17.0	25.0
1910	15.6	24.1	14.5	21.7
1920	13.7	20.6	12.6	17.7
1930	11.7	20.1	10.8	16.3
1940	10.2	16.3	10.4	13.8
1950	8.0	12.3	9.5	11.2
1960	7.3	10.5	9.5	10.1
1970	6.8	9.8	9.5	9.4

Source: Bureau of the Census, *Historical Statistics of the U.S. Colonial Times to 1970*, Bicentennial edition, pt. 1. Washington, D.C.: U.S. Government Printing Office, 1975, p. 59.

In conclusion, then, I have sketched some of the economic and demographic changes that have taken place in the Navajo population over the past century or more. By some criteria economic conditions have not improved significantly, if at all, but mortality rates have declined dramatically, especially since

World War II. This raises the question addressed in the next chapter, namely, what contribution has curative and preventive medicine made to improved mortality relative to the contribution of larger social and economic changes. It shall be suggested that, unlike among the greater U.S. population and those of Western Europe where medical measures were not the major determinants of the decline in mortality, among Navajos the decline was caused largely by such medical measures.

3

Disease Patterns on the Navajo Reservation

MORTALITY rates had already declined substantially by the mid-1950s when the Public Health Service assumed responsibility for services to Indian communities and began to record vital events. Nonetheless, the change in causes of mortality and morbidity that accompanied this decline continued. This transition is illustrated in table 3.1, which shows the proportionate distribution of deaths by cause among Navajos in 1954–1956, 1965–1967, and 1973–1975.

The table shows the rapid decline in deaths from influenza, pneumonia, gastroenteritis and diarrhea, and the dramatic increase in accident mortality. Heart disease increases slightly, but because symptoms and ill-defined conditions still constitute about 20 percent of the diagnoses, it may be that the increase is merely an artifact of better reporting. The pattern of deaths from cancer suggests a certain amount of random fluctuation, and thus is much less certain than the patterns for major diagnostic categories such as accidents and diarrheal and respiratory diseases.

Despite changes since 1955, Navajo mortality still differs from that of the U.S. population in respect of the proportionate contribution of different causes to the overall rate, as the last column in table 3.1 demonstrates. Accidents of all types, particularly from motor vehicles, are far more significant for Navajos than for the population generally. The same is true for influenza and pneumonia, and for gastroenteritis. Cancer and heart dis-

TABLE 3.1
PROPORTIONATE DISTRIBUTION AND ESTIMATED RATES OF MAJOR CAUSES OF MORTALITY, NAVAJO AREA, 1954–1975

	1954–1956[a]		1965–1967[a]		1973–1975[b]		1976 U.S. all races	
	%	Rate per 100,000	%	Rate per 100,000	%	Rate per 100,000	%	Rate per 100,000
Accidents	16.8	118–134	22.9	149–172	31.4	188–220	6.9	43.2
Diseases of the heart	4.2	29–34	6.5	42–49	7.6	46–53	34.5	216.7
Malignant neoplasms	3.4	24–27	7.4	48–56	5.8	35–41	21.0	132.3
Influenza & pneumonia (excluding newborns)	14.2	99–114	8.1	53–61	5.8	35–41	2.8	17.4
Certain diseases of infancy	9.6	67–77	7.4	48–56	3.0	18–21		
Gastritis, enteritis and diarrheal diseases	10.5	74–84	5.6	36–42	1.6	10–11		
Estimated crude death rate per 1,000		7–8		6.5–7.5		6–7		6.3

aUSPHS 1971:27 (includes Hopi reservation)
bUSPHS 1979:94

ease, however, are less significant among Navajos. Interestingly, the Navajo mortality rate from gastroenteritis in 1973–1975 (10 to 11 per 100,000 population) was the same as the rate for the general population in 1940, whereas the Navajo death rate from influenza-pneumonia in 1973–1975 was about the same as the rate for the general population in 1960. By contrast, mortality rates from accidents have been higher among Navajos than they have ever been among the general population from 1900 to the present. Moreover, among Navajos this rate is increasing whereas in the general population it has decreased from about 84 per 100,000 in 1900 to 56 in 1970 (see appendix II).

The impact of contemporary Navajo mortality patterns has been examined by Carr and Lee (1978), who have shown that in 1973 life expectancy at birth was 58.8 for males and 71.8 for females. Eliminating automobile accidents as a cause of death would add 5.17 years of life at birth for men and 2.7 for women; eliminating all other accidents would add 3.13 years of life at birth for men (data for women were not published); eliminating diseases of the circulatory system would add 3.31 years of life for men and 3.70 for women. These patterns differ substantially from those of the U.S. population and illustrate the enormity of the accident problem among Navajos, especially males.

Two other points are worth making. First, life expectancy at one year of age does not differ dramatically from life expectancy at birth for each sex: 59.6 for males and 72.4 for females. This indicates that infant mortality is no longer the major contributor to diminished life expectancy that it once was. Second, infectious diseases do not appear among the five major causes of diminished life expectancy.

Judging from comparative data based upon hospital utilization—that is to say, hospitalized morbidity rather than mortality—infectious and parasitic diseases, accidents, deliveries, and perinatal problems account for most Navajo hospitalizations and are all more significant than in the general population (table 3.2). Neoplasms and circulatory diseases are more significant among the general U.S. population. Hospitalized morbidity is thus congruent with mortality patterns and indicates that Navajos still have disease patterns that are substantially different from the rest of the population. The remainder of this chapter will discuss some of those disease categories in greater detail.

TABLE 3.2

DISCHARGE RATES BY DIAGNOSTIC CATEGORY/10,000 POPULATION

Diagnosis	Navajo 1972	United States Total	United States Western	SDR[†]
Special conditions and exams w/o illness	68.0	15.3	12.5	4.9
Infectious-parasitic	155.1	38.6	29.4	3.7
Perinatal mortality and morbidity	18.8	4.2	5.0	2.6
Symptoms and ill-defined conditions	63.0	28.8	25.8	2.5
Delivery and complications	346.1	200.9	182.6	1.9
Nervous system and sense organs	92.3	59.7	64.0	1.8
Injuries and adverse effects	237.0	159.3	173.3	1.7
Skin and subcutaneous tissue	35.8	25.0	23.2	1.6
Mental disorders	60.9	57.6	53.8	1.4
Endocrine-nutritional-metabolic disorders	23.4	39.4	28.7	0.87
Respiratory diseases	160.9	172.1	152.5	0.85
Congenital anomalies	17.1	17.5	15.5	0.74
Blood and blood-forming organs	7.4	12.6	8.9	0.67
Digestive diseases	78.4	194.7	149.3	0.54
Genitourinary diseases	54.3	159.2	127.6	0.43
Musculoskeletal	20.7	72.0	84.8	0.40
Circulatory diseases	36.1	189.0	159.1	0.37
Neoplasms	23.3	102.8	97.0	0.36
All conditions	1,744.2	1,548.6	1,393.0	1.38
Total N	21,431	31,627,000	4,894,000	

Source: Davis and Kunitz 1978.

[†]SDR = $\dfrac{\text{Number of observed Navajo discharges}}{\text{Number of expected Navajo discharges}}$ = Standardized Discharge Ratio

(Navajo rates standardized to the general United States population)

TUBERCULOSIS

Archaeologists, physical anthropologists, and others interested in paleopathology have argued about the antiquity of tuberculosis in the New World. The most recent evidence suggests it was present in pre-Columbian America (Buikstra 1981). That it became a major scourge after contact with Europeans is said to be the result of the starvation and deprivation that ensued. Unfortunately, the vital data are missing to show the magnitude of its impact on the Navajos until relatively recently. Crude mortality rates per 100,000 population from tuberculosis have been gathered from the beginning of the century to the present (table 3.3).

TABLE 3.3
NAVAJO CRUDE TUBERCULOSIS DEATH RATES PER 100,000 POPULATION

Year	Rate/100,000	Source
1907	175	Hrdlicka 1909:6
late 1930s	386	Thompson 1951:34
1939	300	Navajo Medical News 1940:23
1950	190	Hadley 1955:835
1954–1956*	64.2	TNY 1961:100
1957–1959*	41.2	TNY 1961:100
1966	20.6	USPHS 1971:28
1975–1977*	6.8	May and Broudy, n.d.:23

*average annual rate

The figure given by Hrdlicka for 1907 is somewhat surprising. Rates from other tribes were all several times higher. By way of explanation he wrote:

The natives most free from tuberculosis—the Navaho—occupy an extensive and naturally healthful region, where they live under conditions more nearly aboriginal than those found in any other locality north of Mexico. The tribe no doubt suffers more from tuberculosis than is indicated in the reports of the Indian Office, for the size of the territory and the number of its people make it impossible as yet to obtain exact data. Still, there are many indications that in this tribe the proportion of tuberculosis cases is very small where contact with the whites is restricted. An exception is found among the Navaho on the Hopi reservation, who already show infection to about the same extent as the Hopi themselves. (Hrdlicka 1909:6−7)

Dr. A. M. Wigglesworth, the physician stationed at Fort Defiance, wrote in his annual report in 1905:

The medical aspect of the Navajo does not differ from that of other Indians in general save in degree. Their independence, frugality, and isolation contribute to making them resistant to disease. . . . Tuberculosis is not prevalent but is increasing, and is always fatal when the lungs or meninges are involved. (Commissioner of Indian Affairs 1905:168; see also Brewer 1906)

It is entirely possible that the low rates resulted from many deaths being unrecorded. Hrdlicka mentions this likelihood. What is not clear is whether deaths were underreported more than the population was underenumerated. If they were, then the rates would not necessarily be spuriously low. If, however, the population were overestimated and deaths were underreported, then the reported rate would in fact be much lower than the actual rate. Indeed, the special censuses of 1890 and 1910 evidently did underenumerate Navajos (Johnston 1966a:103−105), but some critics believed that the Bureau of Indian Affairs generally overestimated the population. Hrdlicka's estimates came from the Bureau of Indian Affairs, and it is therefore likely that the numerator (deaths from tuberculosis) was too low and the denominator (population size) too high, leading to a spuriously low rate.

I do not have reliable figures on deaths from tuberculosis between 1907 and 1939. Although the Annual Reports of the Commissioner of Indian Affairs from 1913 through 1920 were more detailed than the material published before or since, the death reports were estimated. Annual tuberculosis and trachoma surveys were undertaken in these years by physicians from the U.S. Public Health Service, but their population estimates for different Navajo reservations, later called agencies, are virtually worthless. The number of individuals examined and of active cases diagnosed are given without information on sampling procedures; and with one exception screening was done by clinical examination. If we are circumspect in interpreting the results (displayed in tables 3.4, 3.5, and 3.6), however, prevalence rates of active cases may be inferred.

Table 3.4 indicates that the rate of active cases was lower for Navajos than for all Indians and that the rate declined each year. The column labeled "Moqui" refers to the Hopis, but it is unclear how many of these individuals were Hopis and how many were Navajos who may have been included in the same survey. Considering the relatively small samples in this latter group, the rates are not likely to have been significantly different from those found among the Navajos. Moreover, as table 3.6 will indicate, the sampling fractions from each Navajo reservation were probably not equal. Thus, combining prevalence rates into one figure for a tribal average would be misleading.

These observations on the comparative prevalence of active cases of tuberculosis receive some confirmation from a survey of tuberculin reactors in several Colorado and New Mexico Indian populations in 1913 (table 3.5). "In all, 1,225 children of school age were inoculated, with 760 positive reactions, a percentage of 64.4" (Secretary of the Treasury 1913:45). The number of children from each tribe is not clear, with the exception of the small number from Cochiti. Moreover, how representative these children were of the school-age population is unclear since, if most of them were students, this would be a biased sample. Finally, the Navajo children tested were most likely from eastern Navajo reservations, while tuberculosis appears to have been most prevalent in the west. Nonetheless, the data provide some evidence that Navajos did not have an extraordinarily high proportion of tuberculin reactors.

Table 3.6 displays prevalence rates of active cases reported from the different Navajo reservations. It should be pointed out that the 1913 figures from the Western Navajo and the 1917 figures from the San Juan Navajo reservations are almost certainly spuriously high. The Western figures are so out of line with figures reported from the following years that it seems best to regard them as an error. The 1917 figures from San Juan report observations on more Indians than were estimated to be living on that reservation. Moreover, the number is so nicely rounded and so much higher than any other sample reported that it seems almost certainly an estimate rather than a valid report.

TABLE 3.4

RESULTS OF TUBERCULOSIS SURVEYS, 1913–1920

Year	NAVAJOS # Examined	# Active tbs	%	MOQUI # Examined	# Active tbs	%	ALL INDIANS # Examined	# Active tbs	%
1913	2,723	396	14.5	1,797	23	1.3	61,201	8,012	13.1
	*(1,982)	(183)	(9.2)						
1915	3,166	267	8.4	900	23	2.5	66,729	7,195	10.8
1916	5,663	222	3.9	612	30	4.9			
1917	11,944	1,665	13.9	1,665	82	4.9			
	*(4,444)	(157)	(3.5)						
1918	missing data						64,272	3,941	6.1
1919	5,340	171	3.2	814	8	0.9	62,756	3,293	5.2
1920	5,910	145	2.4	549	19	3.4	66,718	4,519	6.8

*probably spuriously high rate not included

Source: Annual Reports, Commissioner of Indian Affairs, Washington, D.C.: U.S. Government Printing Office.

TABLE 3.5
PERCENTAGE OF SCHOOL-AGE CHILDREN WITH POSITIVE
TUBERCULIN TESTS BY TRIBE, 1913

Tribe	Percentage of positive reactors	
	Under 11 years of age	Over 11 years of age
Mescalero Apache	63.6[a]	82.3[a]
Jicarilla Apache	68.7	95.5
Southern Ute (Ignacio, Navajo Springs)	72.4	88.8
Southern Ute	75	62.5
Navajo	46	78
Zuni	26.8	55.4
Taos	3.5	1.4
Laguna	44.6	63.2
San Juan, Santa Clara, San Ildefonso, Nambe, Tesuque	70	81
Cochiti	50[b]	44[c]

[a]boys only   [b]2 subjects   [c]9 subjects

With these caveats in mind, it appears that the rates of active cases declined in all populations surveyed except the Western Navajo (including Leupp). The Western Navajo were by far the poorest population in the 1920s, and it is not unreasonable that tuberculosis should have been more prevalent among them. This decline for all but the Western Navajos is difficult to reconcile with the increase in mortality shown in table 3.3, a situation complicated by the fact that the 1939 mortality figures are as bedeviled as those from 1907 by being undercounted by an unknown degree. Of the 154 deaths from tuberculosis recorded in 1939, most were known from hospital records. How many deaths occurred out of hospitals is not known; nor is it known whether the cause of death was accurately recorded. In the late 1930s a physician with many years of experience on the reservation said that where he worked, perhaps 25 percent of deaths were accurately diagnosed and "in the back stretches of the reservation a much smaller percentage" (Joslin 1940:2036). At about the same time, the Phelps-Stokes Fund (1939:82) reported

TABLE 3.6
NAVAJO AGENCIES: ACTIVE CASES OF TUBERCULOSIS

Year	Western Navajo			Leupp			Navajo			San Juan		
	Examined	Active	%	Examined	Active	%	Examined	Active	%	Examined	Active	%
1913	741	213	28.7**	500	46	9.2	1,000	110	11.0	482	26	5.4
1915	621	80	12.9	600	1	0.1	1,500	134	8.9	445	52	11.7
1916	978	77	7.9	700	12	1.7	1,760	60	3.4	2,225	73	3.3
1917	1,191	76	6.4	728	9	1.2	2,525	72	2.8	7,500	1,508	20.0
1918	No data			360	11	3.0	No data			700	10	1.4
1919	1,350	100	7.4	110	8	7.3	2,500	50	2.0	1,380	13	0.9
1920	300	40	13.3	625	42	6.7	2,100	13	0.6	2,885	50	1.7
Total*	5,181	586	11.3	3,623	129	3.5	11,385	439	3.8	15,617	1,732	11.0
	(4,440)	(373)	(8.4)‡				(8,117)			(224)		(2.7)†

Source: Annual Reports, Commissioner of Indian Affaris
*Many of these may be duplicates (cases examined in more than one year).
**possible error
†without 1917 data
‡without 1913 data

that the Navajo Medical Service was unable to provide sufficient data to calculate crude death rates, much less death rates from tuberculosis.

The same study reported that on the basis of skin test (PPD) and X-ray surveys, 900 cases of tuberculosis were estimated to exist on the reservation (Phelps-Stokes Fund 1939:88). With a population of 48,000 to 50,000, the rate of active cases would have been in the vicinity of 1.8 percent, not significantly lower than the 2.4 percent estimated in 1920. Because case-finding methods may have been more thorough in the later period, the rate might have been significantly higher in 1920 than in the 1930s. However, the accurate diagnosis of a minimum of 154 deaths from tuberculosis in 1939 may mean that the tuberculosis problem had not improved over the preceding 30 years. Indeed, in the absence of adequate data, I believe that tuberculosis may have declined in the first two decades of the century, as it did among other Indians (Reifel 1949), and then began to increase again in the third and fourth decades (1920–1939).

I can be more positive about the data after World War II. Mortality declined dramatically, though the causes are not completely clear. The mortality rate for 1950 (190 per 100,000) is a substantial decline from the estimate for 1939. By contrast, estimates of prevalence of active cases in 1948 (Reifel 1949:237) and 1950 were 2 to 3 percent, about what they had been in the late 1930s. These were confirmed by very thorough case-finding surveys in the Many Farms area in the late 1950s (Deuschle 1959).

The decline in mortality between 1939 and 1950 cannot be attributed to antibiotic therapy because, as Deuschle (1959:202) noted, major changes in treatment did not occur until 1952. At that time, a government program of contracting with off-reservation sanatoriums to care for patients with active infectious tuberculosis was established, and the new and potent antituberculous drug, isoniazid, became available. Moreover, BCG vaccination was not in general use on the Navajo reservation until the late 1940s, though controlled trials had been instituted on a number of other reservations in 1936 (Commissioner of Indian Affairs 1946:362; Aronson and Palmer 1946; Aronson 1948; Aronson et al. 1958; Reifel 1949).

With the prevalence of active cases roughly constant and mortality declining, it appears there was a decline in the case fatality rate, just as there may have been an increase in the fatality rate in the 1920s and 1930s. For example, in 1939 there were 154 deaths known and an estimated 900 active cases. If we assume that the number of active cases was actually 1,500 (3 percent of the estimated population), then we obtain a case fatality rate of about 10 percent. If we assume 1,000 active cases, we obtain a rate of 15.4 percent. Indeed, the rate may have been higher if the actual number of tuberculosis deaths was higher than reported in 1939, as seems likely.

Hadley (1955) estimated a population of 69,000 and a tuberculosis mortality rate of 190 per 100,000 in 1950. The number of deaths was therefore 131. If we assume that the proportion of active cases was 3 percent, the upper figure estimated by Deuschle (1959), then there were approximately 2,000 (2,070) such individuals in the population in 1950. Thus, the case fatality ratio was between 6 and 7 percent. The case-fatality ratio may have declined over an eleven-year period prior to the introduction of antibiotics, adequate sanatorium treatment, and the widespread use of BCG vaccinations. I do not believe that underreporting of deaths was worse in 1950 than in 1939. Similarly, the estimation of the active cases was not significantly less accurate in 1939 than in 1950, the earlier estimate having been based upon reasonably sophisticated surveys by Dr. Esmond Long, tuberculosis consultant to the Office of Indian Affairs (Phelps-Stokes Fund 1939:88).

The decline is problematical if we cannot account for it as the consequence of improved medical therapy. Another possible explanation is that the involvement of an estimated 13,000 to 15,000 Navajos in the armed forces and war-related industries during World War II brought about improvements in nutrition and health. Though the reservation economy suffered greatly in the immediate postwar years, emergency supplies may have helped to maintain the nutritional level that had been achieved in the preceding years.

A more likely explanation for the decline in case fatality ratios between 1939 and 1950 is linked to the decline in deaths from influenza and pneumonia which began nationwide in the

late 1930s (Lerner and Anderson 1963:43) and may have occurred on the Navajo reservation as well, as first sulfa drugs and
then antibiotics became available at just this time. Death rates
from tuberculosis were excessively high during the influenza
pandemic in 1919.[1] Indeed, most patients with chronic diseases
continue to have an increased probability of dying during an
influenza epidemic. Therefore, if influenza and pneumonia
were increasingly treatable on the Navajo reservation during the
1940s, mortality from tuberculosis would have declined as those
patients suffering from the disease would have had a greater
chance of surviving episodes of superimposed infections. This
would help explain declining mortality in the face of a constant
prevalence of active cases (i.e., a declining case-fatality rate)
before specific antituberculosis therapy was developed.

The very dramatic declines in mortality from 1950 to 1954–
1956 and 1957–1959 are almost certainly related to improvements in tuberculosis therapy. The decline over the eleven years
between 1939 and 1950 was about 33 percent (from approximately 300 to 200 deaths per 100,000); over the next three or
four years, during which a crash program of treatment was
instituted, the mortality rate dropped another 66 percent (from
190 to 64 per 100,000). Moreover, the tuberculin reactor rate
among school children six to ten years of age declined from 50 to
60 percent in 1950 to 20 percent in 1959 (Deuschle 1959:202).
Miliary and meningeal tuberculosis, common in the late 1940s
and early 1950s, had all but vanished by the late 1950s. Nutritional and health status had not improved so dramatically as to
account for changes of this magnitude, and I believe that specific
medical measures brought about the decline in tuberculosis morbidity and mortality.

It should be pointed out that the changing pattern of tuberculosis mortality among Navajos—a probable decrease from the
early years of the century to about 1920, an increase through the
1920s and 1930s, and an increasingly rapid decline from the
1940s to the present—is very different from the pattern reported for the population of Massachusetts from 1861 and for
the national population from 1900 (see appendix II). In each of
those examples there was a steady decline beginning well before
chemotherapy was introduced in the 1930s.

INFANT AND CHILDHOOD MORTALITY

The Navajo economy seems to have worsened sufficiently in the 1920s and 1930s to have caused an increase in infant mortality, a sensitive indicator of socioeconomic and environmental conditions. Among the Ramah population, infant and early childhood mortality rates increased in the late 1920s and began to decline in the late 1940s (see table 3.7).

TABLE 3.7
INFANT AND EARLY CHILDHOOD MORTALITY RATES OF RAMAH NAVAJOS

Birth cohort group (interval of birth years)	Infant death rate/1,000 live births	Early childhood death ratios per 1,000 survivors (ages 1–4)
1890–1909	60	59
1910–1924	89	126
1925–1939	141	85
1940–1949	133	106
1945–1954	77	68
1950–1959	32	31
1955–1963	43	–

Source: Morgan 1973:287

Once again it must be asked whether the data from Ramah reflect at all accurately the situation of the entire population. Reporting did not become adequate until the 1950s, so it is very difficult to do more than suggest that the Ramah pattern was not unique. The study of census returns from Hopis and Navajos in 1900 cited in chapter 2 clearly indicates that childhood mortality was higher among the former than among the latter (Johansson and Preston 1978). Dr. Breid's comments comparing the two tribes have also been cited previously (Commissioner of Indian Affairs 1905:165).

In the same year as Dr. Breid recorded his observations, Miltona Keith, the field matron at Third Mesa on the Hopi Reservation, wrote; "An unsolved problem is in the feeding of poorly nourished and sickly children. A large percentage of the mortality among the Oraibi babies is on account of poor nutrition" (Commissioner of Indian Affairs 1905:166). Such comments are not recorded about the Navajos. For example, in that same year, Dr. Wigglesworth at Fort Defiance remarked, "Infant mortality is large, especially in summer, and is due to lack of care" (Commissioner of Indian Affairs 1905:168). And according to J. E. Maxwell, the agent at Canyon Diablo (the Leupp Agency),

> The health of the Indians of this reservation during the past year has been generally good, considering the mode of living and the large amount of rain and severe weather. The deaths that have occurred have been mostly among the small children and due generally to exposure in severe weather and lack of proper medical treatment. (Commissioner of Indian Affairs 1905:171)

The general impression is of a harsh life, with infants and children being exposed to a hazardous environment; but starvation and unsanitary living conditions did not impress observers as they did on the Hopi reservation (Kunitz 1974a).

By 1940 one gets quite a different impression. Safran, a physician at the Tuba City Hospital, reviewed all deaths in that facility during fiscal year 1939. Of a total of 40 people who died, 26 were three years and under in age.

> There were two cases of intracranial hemorrhage of the newborn; both infants were admitted shortly after delivery in the hogan and survived only a few days. There was one case of severe second and third degree burns of the body. There were three cases of neglected premature infants each admitted in a state of severe marasmus (emaciation). None of these lived long enough for us to initiate any therapy. There was one case of miliary tuberculosis and two of tuberculosis meningitis. By far the greatest number of deaths (13) were in the group that died of broncho-pneumonia with or without severe diarrhea; but practically always with an underlying chronic state of malnutrition. In many cases the deaths from broncho-pneumonia were really children with longstanding malnutrition or marasmus who were afflicted with an intercurrent infection and eventually succumbed to a terminal pneumonia. There was obviously a very striking difference in response to therapy in this group of pneumonia cases coupled with malnutrition and in the groups of children who resisted similar pathology but who were in a better state of nutrition. In other words, one could not help but gain the conviction in our pneumonia cases among infants and young children that the underlying state of

nutrition was most often the factor which decided the individual response to whatever type of therapy. The treatment of this group of malnourished, very often marasmic infants with pneumonia, was most discouraging and it was not until we started using sulfanilamide in rather heroic dosages that we were, only occasionally, rewarded with a cure. Lastly, there were as many as four deaths in newborns all due to infections of the umbilical cord with peritonitis and sepsis—obviously preventable. (Safran 1940:14)

He remarked further that, "Frequently we see during our routine hospital work, Navajo children, three years old, who weigh as little as 21 or 22 pounds." Indeed, if half the deaths were caused by underlying severe malnutrition, and if malnutrition was a relatively new phenomenon, then it is entirely possible that the infant and childhood mortality rates could have doubled over a period of twenty or thirty years, as seems to have happened at Ramah.

Table 3.8 displays infant mortality rates covering about a forty-year period beginning in the late 1930s. The figure from the late 1930s—318 per 1,000 live births—is remarkably high and was considered by the author a very rough estimate (Thompson 1951:34). It is much higher than rates reported for other tribes in the same study: Papago, 258; Hopi, 180; Sioux, 110. Even more puzzling is the fact that examinations of 151 Navajo children showed them to be in better health than children in any of the other tribes. Thirty-one percent were found to be in good health as compared to only 17 percent of 153 Hopi children (Thompson 1951:34, 139). It is difficult to interpret these data. It is surprising that the tribe with the highest estimated infant mortality was found to have children who were significantly healthier than a tribe with a much lower infant mortality rate. A chi-square test of the differences in results of physical examinations between the two tribes is significant at less than the 0.01 level. Part of the explanation may be found in the way the samples of children to be examined were drawn.

Examining the original sources (Leighton and Kluckhohn 1948:157; Thompson and Joseph 1947:96), we find that the Hopi samples were drawn from First Mesa, said to be very acculturated, and from Oraibi, a traditional village on Third Mesa. Results of the examinations in each Hopi community,

TABLE 3.8
NAVAJO INFANT MORTALITY, 1939–1976

Date	Rate per 1,000 live births	Area	Source
Late 1930s	318.0	Reservation-wide	Thompson 1951:34
1949–51	139.4	Reservation-wide	Hadley 1955
1949–53	131.4	Navajo-Hopi (Ariz.)	USPHS 1957:235
	134.4	Navajo (N.M.)	USPHS 1957:236
Late 1950s	70.0	Many Farms	McDermott et al. 1972
1970	37.0	Reservation-wide	Brenner et al. 1974
	31.5	Reservation-wide	USPHS 1971
1977	17.6	Reservation-wide	USPHS 1979
1977	13.4	Chinle Service Unit	Ibid.
1977	14.0	Crownpoint SU	Ibid.
1977	16.5	Fort Defiance SU	Ibid.
1977	17.9	Gallup SU	Ibid.
1977	13.7	Kayenta SU	Ibid.
1977	8.3	Shiprock SU	Ibid.
1977	27.4	Tuba City SU	Ibid.
1977	41.6	Winslow SU	Ibid.

dichotomized into healthy and unhealthy (table 3.9), reveal no significant difference when subjected to a chi-square test.

Examination results from the three Navajo communities— Shiprock, which contained many acculturated individuals, Ram ah, which was also very close to Anglo settlements, and Navajo Mountain, one of the most remote places on the reservation— were also tabulated as healthy and unhealthy (table 3.10). A chi-square test reveals no differences among them either.

TABLE 3.9
HEALTH STATUS OF HOPI CHILDREN

	Oraibi	First Mesa
Good health	17	9
Unhealthy	74	53

Source: Thompson and Joseph 1947:96

TABLE 3.10
HEALTH STATUS OF NAVAJO CHILDREN

	Shiprock	Ramah	Navajo Mt.
Good health	14	11	16
Unhealthy	58	26	26

Source: Leighton and Kluckhohn 1948:157

Finally, combining all five samples into one table and examining the differences among them, we find a significant difference (chi-square = 10.47, degrees of freedom = 4, $p < 0.05$), which is accounted for by the higher-than-expected number of healthy children at Navajo Mountain. Thus combining the samples within each tribe blurs some interesting distinctions. The Hopi communities, neither of which was in fact remarkably isolated, do not differ from each other or from the Navajo communities that are also not isolated. Moreover, the non-isolated Navajo communities are intermediate between Navajo Mountain and the Hopi communities, not differing significantly from either.

These same health examination data are also presented by age (table 3.11). Although the original studies do not permit putting the results from the two tribes in precisely the same form, a striking difference emerges nonetheless. Among Hopis, a higher percentage of older than younger children were healthy, especially among girls. Among the Navajos, the pattern was the same, only more dramatic. Leighton and Kluckhohn (1948:160) thought that among the Navajos only the most fit survived infancy and childhood. If this was the case, then by the early 1940s the Hopis were able to keep sickly children alive longer than

TABLE 3.11
PERCENTAGE OF THOSE CONSIDERED HEALTHY WITHIN EACH AGE GROUP

	Age			
	5–7	8–10	11–13	14–18
Hopi[a]	boys 7.1	14.3	13.3	7.7
	girls 7.1	14.3	26.7	28.0
Navajo[b]	3	13	37	65

[a]Thompson and Joseph 1947:145
[b]Leighton and Kluckhohn 1948:158

could Navajos, only to have them die at higher rates during adolescence and early adulthood. This interpretation gains support from the estimates of crude mortality rates in this set of studies: 16 per 1,000 for the Navajos and 25 for the Hopis (Thompson 1951:34).

A number of conclusions are suggested by these data. First, even assuming overestimates of Navajo infant mortality, the rate increased during the first four decades of the present century. Second, the rate reported for the Hopis from the late 1930s and early 1940s is compatible with rates presented elsewhere and calculated independently (Kunitz 1974a). Thus by the late 1930s, Navajo infant mortality increased to at least the Hopi rate and perhaps higher. Third, the high rates of Navajo infant mortality were found in the more remote areas of the reservation such as Navajo Mountain. In such places, sickly children were at much higher risk of dying than in communities like Shiprock and Ramah, where increasingly competent medical care was relatively more accessible and where wage work made possible a higher standard of living.

By the late 1940s and early 1950s, the estimated mortality rates for the entire tribe converge with those calculated for the Ramah population, (see tables 3.7 and 3.8). From that time to the present, there has been a steady fall, accounted for primarily by a decline in postneonatal as opposed to neonatal deaths (see table 3.12). More specifically, about 77 percent of the decline in infant mortality is attributable to the reduction in postneonatal mortality and about 23 percent to a reduction in the neonatal rate.

That the determinants of neonatal and postneonatal mortality differ is suggested by analyses of average annual rates (1972–1976) of each by land management district. Simple correlation of postneonatal rates with various measures of economic status and hospital accessibility show that there is a positive relationship ($r = .54, p = .02$) between household size and rate and a negative relationship ($r = -58, p = .01$) between proportion of employed men and rate. That is to say, the larger the average household size and the smaller the proportion of employed men, the higher the postneonatal mortality rate per 1,000 births. A multiple regression provides essentially the same results. The best single-variable model includes proportion of employed men

TABLE 3.12
NEONATAL AND POSTNEONATAL DEATH RATES, 1955–1976, NAVAJO AREA

Year	Deaths/1,000 Live Births Neonatal	Postneonatal	Source
1955	24.9	62.9	USPHS 1971:17
1956	21.0	42.3	Ibid.
1958	20.3	52.4	Ibid.
1959	22.4	29.7	Ibid.
1960	20.8	50.3	Ibid.
1961	18.9	32.0	Ibid.
1962	14.3	33.5	Ibid.
1963	17.0	37.2	Ibid.
1964	14.6	26.1	Ibid.
1965	14.0	32.2	Ibid.
1966	19.3	33.0	Ibid.
1967	15.1	23.6	Ibid.
1970	14.9	16.6	Brenner et al. 1974
1977	8.7	8.9	USPHS 1979
decline in %	65.0	85.8	

and explains 33 percent of the variance. The best two-variable model explains 45 percent of the variance and adds average age of male household head: once employment is controlled, the older the men, the lower the postneonatal rate.

Turning to neonatal rates, a different picture emerges. Distance from hospital is positively correlated ($r=.47$, $p=.05$), and average age of male ($r=-.46$, $p=.05$) and female ($r=-.55$, $p=.02$) household head are negatively correlated with the average annual neonatal death rate. The best multiple regression model contains two variables and explains 59 percent of the variance. It includes distance from hospital and average age of male household head. Once distance is controlled, the older the men, the lower the rate.

In summary, postneonatal rates are best explained by the employment variable and neonatal rates by access to hospitals. In each case, age of male household heads is negatively related to the rate, suggesting that perhaps youth of families is important in explaining the rates of each.

The factors contributing to the decline in infant mortality

that began sometime in the 1940s include improved medical therapy. Writing of the period before the late 1950s when the Cornell-Many Farms Project was in operation, McDermott et al. (1972) observed:

> It is fairly certain (despite the poor quality of the vital statistics) that in the two decades prior to the study, decades in which there were no significant field health services, the overall Navajo infant mortality had been steadily falling from around 150 to 85 per 1,000 live births. The principal identifiable change in that period is the improved services in the six hospitals that are distributed over the 23,000 square-mile area. In addition, an effective technology, available only in the hospital environment, did exist for important segments of the infant disease pattern.

Another factor of major importance is nutritional status. At the Tuba City Hospital in 1939, about 16 of 26 deaths among children three years of age and younger were attributable to marasmus. In a six-month period in 1960–61, three cases of kwashiorkor were treated in the same hospital (Wolf 1961). Subsequently, a study of 4,355 admissions of children below the age of five years at the same hospital in 1963–1967 (Van Duzen et al. 1969) indicated that 616 were suffering from some degree of malnutrition, including 15 cases of kwashiorkor, and 29 of marasmus. Of these 44 children, 16 died (case-fatality rate of 36 percent). The number of deaths from malnutrition was the same during the entire five years 1963–1967 as in the single year 1939.

Since the proportion of deaths that occurred in hospitals almost certainly increased between the late 1930s and the mid-1960s, it is likely that during the early period a considerable number of infants and young children suffering from severe malnutrition died without coming to the attention of the health care system. Thus, the death rate from this cause would have been even higher than the early data would indicate. There is some evidence, then, that the prevalence of malnutrition declined significantly during this period.

No adequate surveys of nutritional status were undertaken before the mid-1950s. At that time, Darby and his colleagues studied two communities in the central part of the reservation, Ganado and Pinon. For the most part, they found nutritional status to be adequate. They specifically searched for cases of kwashiorkor and found none (Darby et al. 1956:75), thus confirming the observations of the physicians at Sage Memorial Hospital in Ganado: "Among the 60,000 records examined nutritional diseases were recorded as follows: pellagra, 10; scurvy, 10; beriberi, 2; rickets, 1; and 'malnutrition,' 97" (Darby et al. 1956:40). A difference in diagnostic acumen is unlikely when severe malnutrition appears, and it is probable that nutritional status was worse on the western end of the reservation than elsewhere, as Van Duzen et al. (1969) suggested.

A second field study of nutritional status, in Greasewood, somewhat to the east of Ganado and Pinon, was carried out in 1968–69 (Reisinger et al. 1972). The results, though not exactly comparable to those of the earlier study, indicated that nutritional status was better than it had been in the mid-1950s.

> Frank, specific malnutritional states were not often found in the younger portion of the population by clinical or laboratory examination. However, low serum levels of specific nutrients were observed in portions of the adult population, though clinical signs of specific nutritional deficiencies were not found. Marginal iron deficiency was demonstrated in all age groups by the high prevalence of low serum iron and low transferrin saturation values. (Reisinger et al. 1972:88)

A small retrospective case-control study done in Shiprock at about the same time of infants diagnosed as suffering from neglect (including several with varying degrees of malnutrition) indicated that the neglected infants were especially likely to have mothers who were single, widowed, or divorced and who came from smaller families than did the controls (Oakland and Kane 1973). A somewhat larger prospective study of the impact of aggressive postnatal follow-up care of infants during the first year of life found that infants receiving special attention did not differ from those receiving routine care with regard to mortality, morbidity, and nutritional status (Rogers et al. 1974). Medical care thus appears to be somewhat less significant than a variety of environmental and social factors in influencing the health of infants at present.

This conclusion is supported by the assessment of McDermott et al. (1972) regarding their accomplishments after five years of delivering primary health care at Many Farms: they observed that they had not effected a reduction in the occurrence of the pneumonia-diarrhea complex, which remained the single greatest cause of illness and death (see also McDermott 1966). This complex affects infants and children particularly and, as a number of studies in developing nations have shown, is intimately related to nutritional status, particularly the phenomenon known as weanling diarrhea (Scrimshaw et al. 1959).

Mortality from gastroenteritis in 1973–1975 was between 11.9 and 14.8 percent of what it had been in 1954–1956, whereas mortality from influenza and pneumonia was between 30.7 and 41.4 percent of the earlier rate. This relatively greater decline in diarrheal than respiratory mortality is unusual. Preston (1976:40) has shown that in non-Western populations, as mortality rates decline to levels achieved earlier by western nations, diarrheal diseases "have tended to gain prominence" in contrast to what is observed in Western nations. That is to say, the overall structure of mortality differs even when age-adjusted death rates are roughly comparable, the difference being accounted for largely by an excess in diarrheal disease.

The Navajo pattern is explained largely by both the decline in prevalence of malnutrition and the increase in homes with running water. In 1960 virtually no Navajo homes on the reservation had indoor water, but in 1978 it was estimated that 57 percent had running water, though not necessarily indoor toilets (Navajo Area Indian Health Service 1979a).[2] Thus, hand washing and clean drinking water had become more common. In a study of the impact of improved sanitary facilities on morbidity patterns in the Hopi village of Moenkopi, diarrhea declined significantly among children in households where water supplies had been improved. Respiratory disease, on the contrary, did not change (Rubenstein et al. 1969). The same is likely to have been the case among the Navajos.

MATERNAL MORBIDITY AND MORTALITY

Women and children benefit most from the epidemiologic transition. In the preceding section I have shown that infant mortality has declined dramatically in the past forty years. The same is true of maternal mortality: from an estimated 1,000 deaths per 100,000 live births in 1940, it has declined to about 29 at present, only slightly more than the rate for the non-Indian population (table 3.13). Elsewhere (Slocumb and Kunitz 1977) it has been suggested that the maternal mortality decline from 1940–1945 to 1946–1953 resulted from a decrease in deaths attributable to sepsis, evidently brought about by increasingly effective treatment as antibiotics became available after World War II. Toxemia and hemorrhage did not decline in those years.

TABLE 3.13
NAVAJO MATERNAL MORTALITY RATES/100,000 LIVE BIRTHS

Year	Rate	Area	Source
Late 1930s, early 1940s	1,000	Reservation-wide	Leighton and Kluckhohn, 1948:15
1948–1950	421	Fort Defiance (hospital deliveries)	McCammon 1951
1968–1969	108.3	Reservation-wide	USPHS 1970*a*, 1970*b*
1972–1979	29.0	Reservation-wide	USPHS 1979:41

TOXEMIA

Toxemia accounts for almost one of three maternal deaths among American Indians. In pregnancy, this disorder is marked by hypertension, proteinuria, and edema. Complications include convulsions (eclampsia), cerebral vascular accidents, liver and kidney failure, consumption coagulopathies (blood clotting), and fetal deaths. Factors thought to influence the incidence of toxemia include maternal nutrition; potentiating diseases such as diabetes, hypertension, and vascular disease; genetic predisposition; and relative maternal-placental insufficiency (twins, primiparas).

The highest incidence of toxemia in the United States occurs among lower socioeconomic groups; populations with inaccessible or inadequate prenatal facilities; and particularly among blacks, in whom essential hypertension is frequent. The incidence of toxemia nationwide is estimated to be between 5 and 7 percent of all deliveries; eclampsia is estimated to occur in 0.12 to 0.26 percent of deliveries. From several studies of Navajos, it is clear that, while declining, rates of toxemia and eclampsia are still somewhat above the national figures (table 3.14).

TABLE 3.14
TOXEMIA AND ECLAMPSIA RATES AMONG NAVAJO WOMEN

| Year | Rate/100 live births | | Area | Source |
	Toxemia	Eclampsia		
1948–1950	13.2	0.41	Fort Defiance	McCammon 1951
1969–1971	15.2	0.32	Fort Defiance	Slocumb and Kunitz, 1977
1972–1973	9.9	---	Navajo Area	Slocumb and Kunitz, 1977
1977–1979	6.8[a]	0	Navajos, Keams Canyon	North et al. 1980
	13.9[a]	0	Hopis, Keams Canyon	North et al. 1980

[a]"pre-eclampsia"

When eclampsia occurs, the rate of maternal mortality soars to between 4 and 6 percent. Toxemia accounted for 19.7 percent of maternal deaths in the United States and for 10.3 percent of maternal deaths in Los Angeles County between 1957 and 1972. Vaughn (1969) reported that among 156 maternal deaths in New Mexico during 1956–1966, toxemia was responsible for 30 percent of those among American Indians. The rate was 35.1 per 100,000, 12.1 times that for Anglo-Americans in the same state. Presumably a rate so excessive compared with rates in other high risk populations reflects either a genetic predisposition or social and health care factors. One such predisposing factor, chronic hypertension, is not common among Navajo women (DeStefano et al. 1979). It has been suggested, however, that the diet, high in salt and starches and low in vitamins and proteins, may be significant. Also of importance may be the lack of prenatal care, which is discussed further below.

SEPSIS

Factors predisposing to sepsis in pregnancy include failure to obtain specimens at an early stage, prolonged rupture of membranes, prolonged labor, pelvic trauma, postpartum hemorrhage, anemia and malnutrition, and lack of early detection and treatment of postpartum fever. Among Navajos at Fort Defiance in 1968–1971, the incidence of postpartum endometritis was 8.8 percent, as opposed to 1.4 percent among whites. McCammon (1951) reported a rate of 6.9 percent at the same hospital in 1950. The higher rate of sepsis among Navajos than non-Indians undoubtedly accounts for the higher rate of mortality from this cause (Vaughn 1969). A lack of preventive services and a lower resistance to the effects of infection owing to anemia and malnutrition may be of etiological importance. I have already noted that the decline in deaths from this latter cause in the 1940s was almost certainly due to the increased availability of antibiotics.

HEMORRHAGE

Hemorrhage in pregnancy is caused by such antepartum conditions as abruptio placenta and placenta previa and by such complications of delivery as ruptured uterus, vaginal and cervical lacerations, and uterine atony resulting in blood loss in excess of 500 cc. Potentiating factors such as anemia and malnutrition result in severe hemorrhage and in maternal mortality when the patient is unable to adjust to the amount of blood lost.

Although maternal deaths from hemorrhage decreased by 75 percent in the general U.S. population from 1940 to 1953, they declined only minimally among Indians during that same period. The rate of maternal death from this cause was 5.4 times higher for Indians than for non-Indians in New Mexico in 1956–1966 (Vaughn 1969). At Fort Defiance in 1968–1971, the incidence of postpartum hemorrhage among Navajo patients was 9.6 percent compared with 5 to 6 percent in the non-Indian population. The combined incidence of abruptio placenta and placenta previa was 2.0 percent, as opposed to 1.1 in the general U.S. population.

Although rates of hemorrhage are difficult to compare from one population and study to another because of variations in diagnostic standards and perceptions of blood loss, it is evident that the incidence is only about two times higher among Indians than non-Indians. This suggests that the high rate of maternal mortality from this cause is related more to the severity of hemorrhage and inadequacy of treatment than to the more frequent occurrence of the complication.

It has already been indicated that one of the major predisposing factors leading to mortality from hemorrhage is anemia. In a survey of the nutritional status of residents of one Navajo community, Reisinger et al. (1972) observed that 20 percent of the nonpregnant, nonlactating women ages seventeen to forty-four had lower than acceptable hematocrits when judged by National Nutritional Survey standards (adjusted for altitude), and 29 percent had lower than acceptable serum iron levels. They noted: "The presence of low hemoglobin levels in the menstruating female population and older males, and low serum iron and TIBC levels, probably indicated low iron intake in these groups."

According to the standards of the National Nutritional Survey, a serum iron of 40 micrograms per 100 ml or more is acceptable. As noted above, 29 percent of the nonpregnant Navajo women had levels below this. By comparison, a World Health Organization survey found the following: serum iron levels lower than 50 mcg per 100 ml in 15 percent of nonpregnant women in rural Israel; 9.5 percent in a rural Hindu community; 51 percent in Vellore, India; 22.1 percent in a rural Mexican community; and 14 percent in Caracas, Venezuela (McFee 1973). Thus, despite the lower level of serum iron defined as acceptable for the Navajos (40 rather than 50 mcg) there is evidence that among nonpregnant Navajo women, iron deficiency is as prevalent as in some underdeveloped areas of the world.

Similar results were observed when transferrin saturation was measured. Of nonpregnant Navajo women ages 17 to 44, 43 percent had levels below 15 percent saturation, the acceptable standard. The comparable figures from other populations were: Israel, 11.4 percent; a rural Hindu community, 25.8 percent; Vellore, 42.5 percent; a rural Mexican community, 28.1 percent; and Caracas, 18.9 percent.

It has already been noted that perhaps the most significant complication of iron deficiency anemia for pregnant women is the inability to withstand hemorrhage. It is also associated with problems for the newborn infant. In a study of Navajo infant mortality, Brenner et al. (1974) found that mothers of infants dying in the neonatal period were anemic more often than were the mothers of infants dying in the postneonatal period or than mothers of a control group of children who survived infancy. Thus, not only is anemia still relatively common, but it seems to be associated with increased maternal complications and neonatal deaths. Moreover, among Navajos, postpartum hemorrhage appears to be associated with an increased prevalence of panhypopituitarism (Prosnitz and Wallach 1967).

HOSPITAL BIRTHS

A gross measure of the utilization of health care is the proportion of infants born in hospitals. Among Navajos there has been a rapid increase in this rate over the past forty years. In the late 1930s, it was estimated that at least 75 percent of births occurred in homes (Boyce 1974; Lockett 1939; Leighton and Kluckhohn 1948). In 1953 Aberle (1966) found that 75 percent of the mothers in Aneth, an isolated Navajo community, had never delivered in hospital, whereas this was true for only 34 percent of the women in Mexican Springs, a less isolated community.

In an unpublished survey of 137 women in the Tuba City area on the western end of the reservation in 1974, it was found that none of the children born before 1929 were delivered in hospital, but 100 percent of those born after 1969 were so delivered. The greatest change occurred between the 1940s and the 1950s (table 3.15).

TABLE 3.15
PLACE OF BIRTH, DELIVERIES OF 137 NAVAJO WOMEN

Year of delivery	Place (in %)		Total no.	No. unknown
	Home	Hospital		
1910–1929	100	0	32	2
1930–1939	91.1	8.9	45	6
1940–1949	69.6	30.4	79	13
1950–1959	21.8	78.2	174	2
1960–1969	2.3	97.7	259	2
1970–1974	0	100	107	0

The increase in the proportion of deliveries occurring in hospital has paralleled the decline in maternal mortality. It also has been accompanied by an increase in the Caesarean section rate. In 1948–1950 at the Fort Defiance hospital there were 17 Caesarean sections per 1,000 deliveries (McCammon 1951); in

1968–1971 there were 78 (Slocumb and Kunitz 1977). The relatively low rate in 1948–1950 is accounted for partially by the equal number of internal versions (babies turned in utero by internal manipulations), a procedure that is generally no longer done.

Age-specific Caesarean section rates calculated for Navajos for the years 1972 to 1978 (table 3.16) show a consistent increase, paralleling that of the nation generally. The increase occurred in all age groups but especially among the 15- to 19-year-olds, which suggests that increasingly it is a discretionary rather than an emergency procedure. This is a distinction to which I shall return in chapter 5 in an analysis of the use of services. To anticipate the discussion there, I shall suggest that discretionary care is most likely to be used by better educated and more highly acculturated people. The following analyses support the hypothesis.

TABLE 3.16
CAESAREAN SECTIONS AMONG NAVAJOS, 1972–1978

Year	N	Age		Rate/1,000 deliveries			
		mean	median	15–19	20–34	35–49	Total
1972	147	27.0	26.0	28	50	50	45
1973	179	25.9	25.0	34	59	56	52
1974	197	24.5	23.0	63	58	47	58
1975	229	24.4	23.0	78	63	68	66
1976	309	25.4	24.0	82	93	115	93
1977	367	25.3	24.0	97	93	144	99
1978	375	25.0	24.0	108	107	132	115

Results of regression analyses using rates of Caesarean sections per 1,000 deliveries for women in different age groups as the dependent variables are presented in table 3.17. Examining first the change in overall rate of Caesarean section per 1,000 deliveries from 1972 to 1976, notice that the best single-variable model includes proportion of income from welfare: the lower the dependence upon welfare, the greater the rate of change. The best two-variable model adds proportion of households with a vehicle: the higher the proportion, the greater the change. The best three-variable model adds proportion of women working

TABLE 3.17
COEFFICIENTS OF DETERMINATIONS, R^2, FOR EACH CONSECUTIVE MODEL:
CAESAREAN SECTIONS

	Independent variables	R^2	Regression coefficients	Standard error
Caesarean section:				
All women, change in	WELF	.2860	−0.037*	0.013
rate/1,000 deliveries	VEHIC	.4349	0.023*	0.009
(1976−1972)	WORKF	.5020	−0.028[n.s.]	0.021
Women 19 and under,	VEHIC	.2474	0.103[n.s.]	0.064
rate/1,000 deliveries	WORKM	.3352	0.063[n.s.]	0.045
Women 20−34	HOGAN	.2349	−0.174*	0.079
rate/1,000 deliveries				
Women 35−49,	HOGAN	.1966	−0.286[n.s.]	0.145
rate/1,000 deliveries				

*$p < 0.05$. All models significant at $p < 0.05$ except the last one.
n.s. = not significant

full time: the higher the proportion, the greater the change.

What we observe, then, is that the change in the rate of Caesarean sections per 1,000 deliveries is strongly related to measures of involvement in the wage economy. Not surprisingly, when we examine the average rate of C-sections within age groups, we find a similar pattern. Among women 19 years of age and younger, the rate of Caesarean sections per 1,000 deliveries is related to the availability of vehicles and the proportion of men working full time. Among women ages 20 to 34 only the one-variable model is significant: the higher the proportion of families living in hogans, the lower the rate of Caesarean sections. Among women 35 to 49, there is no regression model that reaches statistical significance. These results are similar to those for induced abortions and tubal ligations (Temkin-Greener et al. 1981).

There are a number of factors affecting the rates of this procedure: availability of support services, referral patterns, and attitudes toward vaginal delivery after a previous Caesarean section. I have no way of determining whether the increase in rate has had any impact on the well-being of mothers and infants. It would appear that maternal and infant health have improved dramatically over the past forty years, and the consequences of increased surgery—for good or ill—may simply be overwhelmed by the much larger changes created by improved nutrition and prenatal care.

PRENATAL CARE

The utilization of prenatal care is generally associated with improved outcome for both mother and child, though the causal connection may be unclear in some cases, as mothers who avail themselves of those services may be the ones who would experience fewer problems regardless of the services used. Nonetheless, there is some reason to believe that prenatal care does make a difference.

Comparisons of prenatal care data between two groups of Navajos and a New York City population indicate clear differences in utilization of services (table 3.18). The high frequency among Navajos of older patients having borne five or more offspring is apparent. Compared with the New York City data from a mixed white and nonwhite population, however, the difference in parity is far more marked than the age difference, as the Many Farms data show most clearly. Despite this, the proportion of mothers first seen in the third trimester or not at all is much higher among Navajos than among the New York City population.

TABLE 3.18
UTILIZATION OF PRENATAL CARE (IN PERCENT)

Parity, age, and trimester seen	Many Farms 1955–1960[a]	Fort Defiance 1968–1971[b]	New York City 1968[c]
Primipara	8.3	26.4	36.5
Age >35	—	11.5	8.4
Parity >5	38.5	26.4	12.5
Trimester first seen			
first	13.0	22.2	41.8
second	17.0	27.9	36.2
third	23.0	31.6	13.0
none	47.0	18.3	3.3

[a]Loughlin 1962
[b]Slocumb and Kunitz 1977
[c]Kessner 1968

The lack of prenatal care may be reflected in the greater complication rate from toxemia, which may be prevented or modified by early diagnosis and treatment. The severity of hemorrhage may also be modified (less so than the incidence) by the early detection and treatment of iron deficiency anemia. In a study of a mixed Navajo and Hopi population at the Keams Canyon Hospital (North et al. 1980), infants whose mothers had no prenatal care had significantly more newborn complications that those whose mothers had had some care. Moreover, as the number of prenatal visits increased, the proportion of low birthweight infants decreased. Similar results were reported by Brenner et al. (1974) in their 1970 study of Navajo infant mortality.

It can be concluded, then, that the diseases formerly most significant in their impact upon adult mortality appear to have been reduced primarily by medical measures—for example, by the use of antibiotics. Infant and child mortality, in contrast, have declined as a result of less specific changes—for example, from dietary improvements, increasing availability of domestic water supplies, and the like.

HEART DISEASE

Turning now to man-made and degenerative diseases, in the general United States population, the epidemiologic transition has been accompanied by an increase in cardiovascular disease. To date, such a development has not occurred among the Navajos, a population notable for their lack of circulatory disorders. It might be expected that rheumatic heart disease, at least, would have a high incidence among Navajos since it is the result of streptococcal infections and thus has a very different etiology than ischemic heart disease. Considering the poverty of the Navajos, the general prevalence of respiratory infections, and the relative inaccessibility of medical care, streptococcal infections and hence rheumatic heart disease would be expected to be higher than that found in the non-Indian population.

In fact, this is not the case. Clinical studies of the prevalence of rheumatic heart disease among American Indian school children in the early 1930s, before the development of antibiotic therapy, indicated the following: among Crow, Shoshone, and Arapahoe children living on reservations in Wyoming and Montana, rheumatic cardiac damage was about twice that found in Anglo school children. Among Navajos, the prevalence rate was slightly lower than among Anglos (1.9 versus 2.2 percent). Among Pimas and Papagos in southern Arizona, the rate was only 0.5 percent (Paul and Dixon 1937). Some conflicting data, however, have been published. Smith (1957) estimated that from 1948 to 1952 slightly more deaths from rheumatic heart disease occurred among Navajos than would have been expected on the basis of rates for the white population of the United States (for men 5 instead of 1.8–2.0; for women 3 rather than 2.0–2.2). These numbers are sufficiently small that it is difficult to be impressed that the rates are wildly out of line. In addition, a more recent review of hospital records from 1962 to 1977 (Coulehan et al. 1980) indicates that attack rates of acute rheumatic fever were not impressively different among Navajos and several non-Indian U.S. populations. The evidence is reasonably consistent, therefore, in indicating that rheumatic heart disease has not been and is not now a major cause of morbidity and mortality.

The relative absence of ischemic heart disease has been even more fascinating to investigators. As Fulmer and Roberts (1963: 740) suggest, this is so because:

> In most less developed societies where coronary heart disease rates are low, the amount of saturated fat in the diet is also relatively low. Navajos, however, have been cited as an exception because their intake of fat has been said to be equal to or even higher than that of the general population in the United States.

There is no doubt that ischemic heart disease is rare among Navajos. Studies of autopsies (Hesse 1964; Streeper et al. 1960), death certificates (Smith 1957), hospitalized patients (Streeper et al. 1960; Sievers 1967; Gilbert 1955), and communities (Fulmer and Roberts 1963) all agree that while coronary artery disease is not unknown, it is unusually rare when comparisons are made with the general population of the United States.

In their study of the Many Farms community, Fulmer and Roberts (1963:749) considered the various risk factors closely associated with the incidence of coronary heart disease in Framingham studies. These included "the distribution of blood pressure, serum cholesterol, and electrocardiographic evidence of left ventricular hypertrophy." Subsequent analyses of data from Framingham suggested that psychosocial stress and type A behavior were also related to coronary heart disease (Haynes et al. 1978*a*, 1978*b*; Haynes, Feinleib, and Kannel 1980).

Blood pressure levels were found to be low among the Many Farms population (Fulmer and Roberts 1963), confirming previous observations (Cohen 1953; Darby et al. 1956). Subsequent surveys of Navajos indicate that hypertension continued to be rare on the reservation (Reisinger et al. 1972; DeStefano et al. 1979) and that blood pressure levels increased when migrants to an urban area were reexamined after they had left the reservation (Alfred 1970). While there is agreement that men tend to have higher blood pressure than women and that obesity increases the risk of hypertension, there is some uncertainty regarding the significance of degree of acculturation. Thus, although the study of off-reservation migrants suggests that acculturation and elevated blood pressure are related, the one study of reservation Navajos that attempted to measure acculturation found no relationship to blood pressure (DeStefano et al. 1979). In this same study, alcohol use was found to be related to elevated blood pressure. However, no data were collected regarding drinking style (occasional versus binge drinking, for instance), so it is very difficult to know what this finding signifies. Finally, in this same study, young Navajo men (20 to 30 years of age) had higher prevalence rates of elevated blood pressure than any other Navajo group and higher rates than either blacks or whites of the same age and of either sex. It is not clear how representative the study group was of the reservation population of this age and sex, but it is conceivable that as this cohort ages, an increase in coronary heart disease and cerebrovascular accidents will be observable.

A second risk factor associated with coronary artery disease is serum cholesterol level. Fulmer and Roberts (1963) observed that the subjects at Many Farms had lower serum cholesterol levels than non-Indian subjects; similar observations have been made by other investigators as well (Page et al. 1956; Kositchek et al. 1961). Why cholesterol levels are lower among Navajos is not clear. Small and Rapo (1970) have speculated that it may be related to the high rate of cholesterol gallstones found among Navajos and other southwestern Indians.

It is obvious that the hepatic cell excretes cholesterol both into the bile as free cholesterol and into the circulation as lipo-proteins. Under normal circumstances there is a balance between cholesterol excretion into bile and into plasma so that the bile is less than saturated with cholesterol. Since the serum cholesterol of these patients is not elevated, and since the Indians, in general, have little atherosclerosis and a high prevalence of gallstone diseases, it is tempting to suggest that the balance between bile and serum release of cholesterol by the hepatocyte is tipped toward bile. (Small and Rapo 1970: 57)

With respect to other risk factors, Fulmer and Roberts (1963) found no evidence of a high prevalence of left ventricular hypertrophy. Nor has obesity been known to be terribly common among Navajos (unlike among the Pimas and Papagos), though several studies suggest that women are more likely to be overweight than men (Reisinger et al. 1972; Fulmer and Roberts 1963; DeStefano et al. 1979). Smoking is also infrequent among Navajos (Fulmer and Roberts 1963; Sievers 1968; DeStefano et al. 1979); and, as for stress, there are no studies of which I am aware that would allow us to say that Navajos experience more or less than non-Navajos. Indeed, low rates of coronary heart disease are sometimes attributed to low stress levels, though other studies attribute high rates of so-called social pathologies (to be discussed below) to high levels of stress. The same lack of data applies to the striving and anxious so-called Type A behavior, though casual observation suggests that it is less common among Navajos than non-Navajos. Finally, with regard to exercise it is generally said that Navajos are less likely to be sedentary than non-Indians.

There is no evidence to indicate that the rate of myocardial infarctions has increased during the 1970s. One hundred and forty-six hospitalizations of men with this diagnosis and 46 of women occurred during the seven fiscal years 1972 to 1978, an average of 27 cases per year with a range of 20 to 42. During these seven calendar years, there were 93 deaths among men from this cause, 24 among women. The median age at death was between 60 and 64 for men; for women it was 70 to 74. The average annual mortality rate was thus about 12 to 14 per 100,000, compared with 158.7 per 100,000 for the white population of the United States in 1976.[3]

THE "SOCIAL PATHOLOGIES"

MOTOR VEHICLE ACCIDENTS

Earlier in this chapter I showed that automobile and other accidents have increased in both absolute and relative significance since the 1950s. However, more has been written about coronary artery disease among Navajos—a disease remarkable for its absence—than about accidents because the former is more likely than the latter to affect those who pay for and do research. The result is that little is known about the accident phenomenon.

The earliest epidemiologic data concerning accidents among the Navajo come from the Many Farms area in 1957–1962 (Omran and Loughlin 1972). Accidental deaths (10 in all) were responsible for 15.4 percent of all deaths. "The leading cause of accidents were domestic injuries, followed by injuries due to sharp instruments that the average Navajo uses in everyday life" (Omran and Loughlin 1972:17). In addition to environmental hazards, the authors argued that psychosocial factors were also significant.

> As a people in transition, the Navajos exhibit many insecurities and inabilities to cope with their changing way of life. This has resulted in a great deal of stress, violence, alcoholism, undisciplined children and social maladjustment. It is generally assumed that the relatively high rate of accidents associated with alcohol and violence is symptomatic of deeper seated social disorders among the Navajos. Drinking was associated with at least five of the fatal accidents, and with the more serious injuries, especially those inflicted by others, as well as a number of motor vehicle accidents. (Omran and Loughlin 1972:18)

A subsequent study based upon hospital records in 1966–1967 showed the Navajo accident death rate to be 104.2 per 100,000—that is, 1.8 times greater than the rate for the U.S. population (58 per 100,000). The rate for Navajo males was 160.6, as opposed to 48.9 for females (relative risk 3.3). Navajo males 25 through 34 had the highest incidence of treated accidental injuries, while males above the age of 65 had the highest death rate from accidents. Motor vehicle accidents were responsible for almost half (48.2 percent) the accidental deaths but accounted for only about 20 percent of the total number of accidents recorded (Brown et al. 1970). It must be emphasized that this was a study of hospital records; thus, people who died before getting to hospital would not necessarily have been included, which probably accounts for the lower reported death rate than that presented previously.

The most recent study of accidents on the Navajo reservation was concerned only with fatal motor vehicle accidents and was based upon a review of police reports (Katz and May 1979). Deaths per 100 million vehicle-miles per year were calculated for various reservation roads between 1973 and 1975. There was some evidence that although the rate dropped from the beginning to the end of the period—presumably as a result of the oil embargo and reduced speed limits—they remained substantially higher than those observed on other roads in New Mexico and Arizona as well as in the United States generally. It was also observed that depending on the type of accident (single or multiple vehicle), the proportion of drivers without valid driver's licenses ranged between 16 and 33 percent. Finally, according to the investigating officers, alcohol was involved in between 41 and 46 percent of accidents (again depending on type). Comparisons made with non-Indians in this study are regarded as misleading since the latter are almost certainly tourists who would differ in numerous ways from the local non-Indian population, but it is worth pointing out that the estimates of alcohol involvement appear low when compared with rates as high as 77 percent from studies of non-Indian populations (Katz and May 1979:66).

The problem of estimating alcohol involvement is a significant one. The conventional wisdom is that Indians drink a lot and therefore have high rates of numerous types of accidents. The only other data I have found bearing upon this point are displayed in table 3.19, a tabulation of the percentage of accidents of different types that, according to the attending professional, were alcohol-related. Almost 20 percent of automobile accidents were thought to involve alcohol use. Comparable data were not collected from non-Indian accident victims, but on the face of it the figures are not remarkably high. Thus the relationship between alcohol use and accidents is unclear. In a previous study of Navajo criminal homicide, it was found that people who had committed homicide did not have any greater prior involvement with alcohol than a control group who had not committed

TABLE 3.19

ALCOHOL-RELATED ACCIDENTS* AS A PERCENTAGE OF
TOTAL ACCIDENTS, NAVAJO AREA, 1972

Type of Accident	Percentage alcohol-related
Motor vehicle	19.5
All other	2.3
Falls	2.1
Cutting, piercing objects	3.2
Suicide attempts	17.9
Injuries purposely inflicted by others	28.7

*treated on an outpatient basis
Source: USPHS 1973

homicide. Nonetheless, the assumption of a causal link between alcohol use and rates of violence is almost invariably made, followed by another assumed causal connection between the stress of acculturation and high rates of alcohol use. The same relationship has been presumed between automobile (and other) accidents and the stress of social change, but as yet there are no data to support or reject the hypothesis.

During the decade of the 1970s, deaths from automobile accidents did not increase (table 3.20), and hospitalizations remained about constant (though average length of hospital stay declined, as it did for all causes; see chapter 5).

Table 3.21 displays age- and sex-specific mortality rates from this cause for Navajos and white Americans. Several points are of interest. Most obviously, the rates for Navajo men and women

TABLE 3.20

NAVAJO MOTOR VEHICLE ACCIDENT DEATHS BY YEAR

Year	Number
1972	146
1973	188
1974	129
1975	161
1976	162
1977	145
1978	131

TABLE 3.21

AVERAGE ANNUAL MOTOR VEHICLE ACCIDENT MORTALITY RATE, 1972–1978
(RATE PER 100,000 POPULATION)

	Navajos*			Whites, 1976		
	Males	Females	Total	Males	Females	Total
<1				6.8	8.4	7.6
1–4				11.4	8.4	9.9
5–14				10.5	6.4	8.5
<10	31.9	29	30.5			
10–14	32.3	11	21.7			
15–24	287	78	176	66.4	20.5	43.7
25–34	392	93	230	37.9	10.4	24.2
35–44	225	88	150	26.3	8.9	17.4
45–54	202	72	134	24.3	9.2	16.5
55–64	249	31	137	24.8	10.8	17.4
65–74				29.5	15.0	21.3
75–84	201	38	130	50.8	21.6	32.5
>85				53.7	14.6	26.9
Total	164	53	106	32.5	12.1	22.1

*Based upon high population estimates. Use of low estimates results in rates as much as 15 percent higher than those in the table.

are much higher than for whites of each sex. Moreover, among non-Indians there is a bimodal curve with peaks in the 15–24 and 75–84 age groups. Among Navajos there is a single peak in the 25–34 age group.

When average annual motor vehicle accident mortality rates among land management districts were analyzed by multiple regression, the best model contained a single variable, average distance to a hospital providing surgery, and explained 51 percent of the variance: the greater the distance, the lower the rate. A similar analysis with average annual hospitalization rate due to motor vehicle accidents as the dependent variable contained the same independent variable and explained 30 percent of the variance: again, the greater the distance from surgery, the lower the rate. I am inclined to explain this as a function of the fact that hospitals offering surgery are in the most densely settled areas with the heaviest traffic. It is unlikely that motor vehicle accident fatalities would go unreported in remote areas of the reservation.

With regard to accident mortality rates, a number of other models are significant. However, the only other independent variable that achieves significance is average age of male household head, which is negatively related and adds 7 percent to the variance explained. Considering the age- and sex-specific rates reported in table 3.21, it should not be surprising that in communities where average age is greater, motor vehicle accident mortality rates are lower.

Thus, mortality from motor vehicle accidents is high at all ages; it peaks in the 25–34 group; and rates are highest in communities where traffic is heaviest and the population is youngest. Police and medical data regarding the significance of alcohol in accidents are equivocal. It appears, however, that the extraordinarily high rates cannot be entirely explained by drunken driving. Inexperienced drivers, risk-taking behavior, poorly maintained vehicles, and the great distances many people drive each year may all contribute.

Finally, it is clear that accidents are the most important explanation of the differences in crude mortality rates among land management district populations. In a multiple regression analysis in which several socioeconomic measures and disease-specific death rates were entered as independent variables, the crude automobile accident mortality rate explained 78 percent of the variance in the crude death rate, and mortality rates from all other accidents added another 12 percent to the variance explained. Thus, 90 percent of the variance in crude death rates is explained by accident mortality rates.

ALCOHOLIC CIRRHOSIS

One of the most widely used measures of alcohol consumption is mortality from cirrhosis of the liver. A study using data from the mid-1960s concluded that Navajos did not have higher rates than the general U.S. population; that men had higher death rates than women but lower case-fatality rates; and that cirrhosis was observed most frequently in border areas where alcohol was readily obtained (Levy and Kunitz 1974).

Mortality data from 1972 to 1978 generally support these observations. Over these seven years there were 181 deaths from cirrhosis of all types, an average of about 26 per year with a range from 18 to 33. Table 3.22 displays average annual age- and

TABLE 3.22
CIRRHOSIS: AVERAGE ANNUAL MORTALITY RATE, 1972-1978
(RATE PER 100,000 POPULATION)

	Navajos*			Whites, 1976		
	Male	Female	Total	Male	Female	Total
<10	0	0	0	0	0	0
10-14	0	0	0	0	0	0
15-24	3.1	.9	2.0	.2	.1	.2
25-34	62	28	44	3.2	1.3	2.3
35-44	103	58	79	17.8	8.1	12.9
45-54	46	47	47	43.3	20.4	31.5
55-64	52	31	42	65.4	28.7	46.1
65-74 ⎫				65.6	25.8	43.1
75-84 ⎬	23	33	28	46.5	20.5	30.3
>85 ⎭				31.0	13.7	19.2
Total	21.8	14.7	18.1	18.9	9.3	14.0

*Based upon high population estimates. Low estimated population based upon preliminary counts from the 1980 census would result in rates 15 percent higher.

sex-specific mortality rates for Navajos and whites. Notice that the total rates for men in each group are essentially the same though age-specific patterns differ. Navajo men have rates that peak in the 25-34 age group, whereas white men have rates that peak in the 55-64 and 65-74 age groups. Moreover, Navajo women have higher rates than white women. It is this last figure that accounts for much of the difference in overall rates between the two populations.

Mortality from cirrhosis has increased both in the general U.S. population (see appendix II) and among Navajos. It is therefore difficult to find an especially unique pattern among the latter, though it appears that, as suggested earlier, Navajo women who drink may still be at higher risk of developing serious problems than are non-Navajo women.

The number of cases of cirrhosis is not large enough to calculate rates for analysis by multiple regression. Instead I have aggregated land management districts into IHS service units, calculated the observed distribution of deaths, and compared that with what would have been expected based upon the population distribution (table 3.23). This is similar to the analysis performed in the earlier study.

TABLE 3.23
DISTRIBUTION OF DEATHS FROM CIRRHOSIS

Service unit	Observed cases	Expected
Tuba City	19	14.7
Kayenta	4	16.7
Winslow	11	11.4
Shiprock	37	38.6
Chinle	13	22.4
Fort Defiance	29	32.2
Gallup	55	27.7
Crownpoint	13	17.4
Total	181	181

$X^2 = 42.23$
$d.f. = 7$
$p < .01$

It is clear that the major contribution to X^2 is accounted for by the much lower-than-expected number of cases in the isolated Kayenta Service Unit and the much higher-than-expected number in the Gallup Service Unit. These results are similar to those observed among hospitalized cases in the mid-1960s and suggest that access to alcohol contributes significantly to the distribution of cases observed.

HOMICIDE

In a previous publication on Navajo criminal homicide using data from 1956 to 1965, average annual rates of 4.5 to 5.3 per 100,000 were calculated. These data were obtained from police records and pertained only to criminal homicide, which includes murder in the first and second degree as well as voluntary manslaughter. Accidental and justifiable homicide and involuntary manslaughter were not included in the analysis or computation of rates (Levy et al. 1969). The figures reported in this section, by contrast, are derived from death certificates, and thus are not comparable to those in the earlier study since they include all homicides without regard to the definition of the act in the eyes of the police and the courts.

Moreover, that earlier study, because it was based upon complete case reports, provided data on both offenders and victims, their relationship, and the circumstances surrounding the event, including involvement of alcoholic beverages. The data used here cannot provide that same richness of detail and only pertain to characteristics of victims: age, sex, and place of residence.

The early study showed that criminal homicide rates were no higher among Navajos than among whites or blacks. In addition, there was evidence that: the rate had not changed significantly during the reservation period; alcohol use did not seem to be causally related to homicides or to the degree of violence of the act; the typical offender was a man in his late thirties who killed his wife and then committed suicide; offenders did not have arrest records that differed from a group of controls, suggesting that there was not a subculture within the population with a history of criminal behavior which increased the probability of committing a homicide; and there was no regional variation in the distribution of homicides. Finally, in contrast to white and black victims, among Navajos, women were more likely to have been victims, a result explained by the fact that homicides resulted from family quarrels and sexual jealousy significantly more frequently than in the other two populations.

Table 3.24 displays average annual age- and sex-specific homicide rates for Navajos and the white population of the United States during the 1970s. Notice that the Navajo rates are higher for each age and sex group and that the rate for males is more than three times as high as that for females. For Navajo males, the rates reach a high plateau between ages 15 and 54; among women between 25 and 54. Among non-Indian males, the rates peak in the 25–34 and 35–44 age groups and then decline quite rapidly. Among non-Indian women there is no peak but rather a constant relatively low level across all age groups.

As noted above, in our study of criminal homicide, no regional variation in distribution was observed. From a comparable analysis of all Navajo homicides between 1972 and 1978 (table 3.25), it is evident that there is no significant difference between the observed and expected distributions, though there is some indication that there were fewer cases than expected in the Kayenta Service Unit.

TABLE 3.24
NAVAJO AVERAGE ANNUAL HOMICIDE RATES, 1972–1978
(PER 100,000 POPULATION)

	Navajos*			Whites, 1976		
	Males	Females	Total	Males	Females	Total
<1				3.9	4.0	3.9
1–4				1.7	1.6	1.6
5–14				.9	.7	.8
<10	2.0	3.3	2.7			
10–14	6.7	1.2	3.9			
15–24	43.2	5.7	23.5	10.6	3.6	7.1
25–34	50.7	14.8	31.2	14.2	3.6	8.9
35–44	48.1	16.7	30.9	13.6	3.2	8.3
45–54	53.3	15.8	33.4	9.6	2.8	6.1
55–64	19.2	4.5	11.6	7.3	2.2	4.6
65–74 ⎫				5.8	2.2	3.8
75–84 ⎬	32.7	4.8	18.9	5.5	3.8	4.4
>85 ⎭				5.5	4.1	4.6
Total	25	7	15.6	8.3	2.7	5.4

*Based upon high population estimates. Use of low estimates from the 1980 census
would result in rates 15 percent higher.

TABLE 3.25
REGIONAL DISTRIBUTION OF HOMICIDES, 1972–1978

Service unit	Observed	Expected
Tuba City	12	12.6
Kayenta	3	14.3
Winslow	11	9.8
Shiprock	40	33.2
Chinle	19	19.3
Fort Defiance	32	27.8
Gallup	28	23.9
Crownpoint	11	14.9
Total	156	155.8

$X^2 = 12.82$
$d.f. = 7$
$p > .05$

SUICIDE

In a study of Navajo suicides between 1954 and 1963, Levy (1965) observed that the average annual rate of 8.3 per 100,000 was not extraordinarily high when compared with rates from other southwestern tribes, the surrounding states, and the general U.S. population. He also observed that in comparison with figures obtained before 1945, there appeared to be a shift among Navajos to an increase of suicides among younger individuals. In addition, males committed suicide more than 13 times more frequently than females; the act was often associated with homicide; there appeared to be no regional variation; and it seemed to have been done impulsively, without advance preparation, and in a setting of domestic strife.

Unlike the previous study of criminal homicide, the records from the early suicide study are more nearly comparable to the data from 1972–1978, save for the possibility that reporting may have become more complete in recent years. From a comparison of age-specific rates in 1954–1963 and 1972–1978 (table 3.26), it is clear that they have generally increased but that the earlier observed pattern of a peak in the 25–39 age groups persists. The peak in the later period is, however, both higher and broader.

The increase is not unique to the Navajos (see appendix II). Table 3.27 displays age- and sex-specific rates for Navajos and the white population of the United States. There are several noteworthy points. First, the crude suicide rates of Navajos and the general population do not differ significantly. Second, Navajo men still kill themselves at a higher rate than Navajo women, but the difference in order of magnitude is now about half what it was in 1954–1963 (6 times rather than 13 times as great). Third, the age pattern still differs from the general U.S. population, with higher rates being observed among the latter group at older ages.

No regional variations were observed in the 1954–1963 period, though data were not presented. Table 3.28 displays the patterns in 1972–1978. Unlike the distribution of homicides, that of suicides does differ significantly from what would have been expected on the basis of population distribution. The major contribution to chi-square is made by the greater-than-expected numbers in the Gallup and Chinle areas and the lower-than-expected number in the Kayenta area.

TABLE 3.26
Navajo Average Annual Age-Specific Suicide Rates,
1954–1963 and 1972–1978 (rates/100,000)

Age	1954–1963	1972–1978*
< 10	0	0
10–14	.9	0
15–19	4.9	18
20–24	9.8	39
25–29	25.6	46
30–34	20.2	38
35–39	32.0	27
40–44	3.2	22
45–49	7.7	24
50–54	8.7	11
55–59	5.3	4
60–64	2.4	14
> 65		14
Total	8.3	14.4

*Based upon high population estimates. Use of low estimates would result in rates 15 percent higher.

DISCUSSION

Of the so-called social pathologies, only accidents contribute significantly to overall mortality patterns. Cirrhosis, suicide, and homicide, while scarcely negligible, are important more as indicators of social processes than as major contributors to mortality. In all four instances, however, an important point stands out: men in their twenties and thirties have the highest rates of mortality. Recall also that this group has the highest prevalence of hypertension.

Previous studies have suggested that this age-sex category may be the focus of special difficulties for several reasons. First, in a traditionally matrilineal and matrilocal society, young men are marginal to the wife's kin group. The high prevalence of domestic conflict noted in earlier studies supports this possibility. Second, these are the people especially exposed to the vagaries of an unstable wage economy. Third, numerous observers have remarked on the emotional lability and impulsiveness of Navajo

TABLE 3.27

SUICIDE RATES PER 100,000, NAVAJOS AND U.S. WHITE POPULATION

Age	Navajo average annual rate* 1972–1978			Whites, 1976		
	Male	Female	Total	Male	Females	Total
< 1	0	0	0	0	0	0
1–4	0	0	0	0	0	0
5–14	0	0	0	.7	.2	.5
15–24	44	10	26	19.2	4.9	12.1
25–34	82	10	43	23.7	8.6	16.2
35–44	48	6	25	23.6	11.0	17.2
45–54	39	0	18	27.7	13.8	20.5
55–64	19	0	9	31.6	12.1	21.3
65–74				36.2	8.9	20.7
75–84	23	5	14	45.6	7.8	22.0
> 85				49.9	5.8	19.8
Total	25.6	4.0	14.4	19.8	7.2	13.3

*Based upon high population estimates. Use of low estimates would result in rates 15 percent higher.

TABLE 3.28

REGIONAL DISTRIBUTION OF SUICIDES, 1972–1978

Service unit	Observed	Expected
Tuba City	11	11.7
Kayenta	5	13.2
Winslow	8	9.0
Shiprock	24	30.7
Chinle	26	17.8
Fort Defiance	30	25.6
Gallup	33	22.0
Crownpoint	7	13.8
Total	144	143.8

$X^2 = 19.91$

$d.f. = 7$

$p < .01$

men (e.g., Levy 1965), the sources of which are not entirely clear. Fourth, as noted in chapter 1, mechanisms of social control among former pastoralists may be less institutionalized than among sedentary agriculturalists, the result being that in the reservation setting aggressive acting-out behavior may be rather marked. The high rates of accidental death and homicide lend some support to this observation.

The regional distribution of these causes of death is also somewhat similar. For suicide and deaths from cirrhosis and motor vehicle accidents, the highest rates are observed in the area near Gallup, New Mexico, and the lowest rates in the remote Kayenta area. Even homicides tend to be lowest in the latter area. Unfortunately, the available data do not include information on migration, so it is impossible to determine whether those who died in the Gallup area were recently arrived or native to the area. As Gallup is one of the most rapidly growing areas on the reservation, it is as reasonable to hypothesize that those who died were migrants as that they were locals. Thus the significance of regional variations is not entirely clear.

Furthermore, although age and sex distributions of the populations in each service unit and land management district are unavailable, there is reason to believe, as chapter 2 indicated, that areas with wage work have younger populations. As these four causes of death occur most frequently in young adult men, it may be that age-adjusted rates, if they could be calculated, would not differ from one place to another on the reservation. Considering the paucity of population data, it may be most reasonable to conclude that the high rates in the Gallup area may result from the most vulnerable segments of the population being exposed to conditions with which they have not been prepared to cope.

REGIONAL VARIATIONS IN THE STRUCTURE OF MORTALITY

So far I have examined mortality piecemeal, one cause at a time. In this section I shall consider contemporary patterns of causes across the reservation, once again using the biplot for a multivariate analysis. Lack of adequate age and sex data at the district level complicate the analysis, forcing me to use crude rates and infer the importance of the structure of the population.

It has already been noted that mortality patterns vary with level of economic development. In general, man-made and degenerative diseases increase in relative importance as economic development increases. I have shown that reservation-wide, this has happened over the past several decades in response both to improvements in medical care and to economic and social changes. I shall now examine the patterns synchronically to determine if the expected variations occur among populations of different land management districts. The expectation is that man-made and degenerative causes will be high in the economically more developed areas and infectious diseases will be high in the less developed areas.

Figure 3.1 is a biplot of the crude rates of death for the most significant causes, along with several variables that measure degree of involvement in the wage economy. Examining first the vectors representing the variables, it is clear that crude rates of all causes of mortality considered separately are positively correlated with one another and with the crude mortality rate. They are inversely correlated with degree of dependence upon welfare and with average distance from the nearest hospital. That is, where mortality rates are high, dependence upon welfare is low and distance from the nearest hospital is also low. Neonatal and postneonatal mortality rates are unrelated to the other measures of mortality.

Though there are relationships between the mortality and economic variables, they are not equally strong in all cases. The crude rate of deaths from circulatory diseases is most strongly positively correlated with the proportion of men working full-time and the proportion of income from wage work and inversely correlated with proportion of income from welfare. The crude death rate and death rates from accidents and gastrointestinal diseases are highly positively intercorrelated, less strongly positively correlated with the wage work variables, and strongly inversely related to the welfare variable. Crude death rates from respiratory and infectious and parasitic diseases and symptoms and ill-defined conditions are very highly positively correlated with one another, unrelated to the wage work vari-

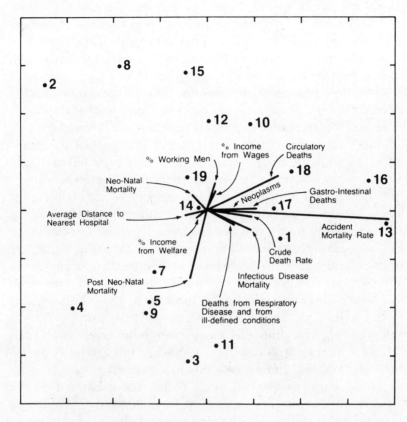

FIGURE 3.1
BIPLOT DISPLAY OF MORTALITY AND ECONOMIC VARIABLES BY LAND
MANAGEMENT DISTRICT, 1970s

ables, and somewhat weakly negatively correlated with the proportion of income from welfare. These last three mortality variables are weakly related to the postneonatal mortality rate and
inversely related to the neonatal mortality rate. Thus, while all
causes of death beyond infancy are in fact closely related, there is
a tendency for circulatory disease deaths to be more positively
correlated with measures of involvement in the wage economy
than are deaths from infectious diseases.

Turning now to the distributions of land management districts (see fig. 2.2), it is apparent that crude rates of all forms of
mortality (except neonatal and postneonatal deaths) are high in

the eastern (district 13) and southeastern portions of the reservation (16, 17, and 18). (District 1 in the northwest and district 10 in the central part also have high rates.) Eastern districts 12 and 15, however, while above average in terms of wage work, have relatively low mortality populations. Thus, the relationship between involvement in the wage economy and deaths from manmade and degenerative diseases is not clear-cut. Districts 3, 4, 5, 7, 9, and 11 in the southwestern and central part of the reservation, by contrast, are above average in post-neonatal mortality rates and below average in involvement in the wage economy.

Postneonatal mortality is the category of mortality most clearly related to economic patterns. As already noted, causes of death involving adults are not as obviously related to economic variables, though populations in which all causes of death are above average tend to be below average in their dependence upon welfare. This is most obvious in the case of deaths from circulatory diseases, which are most strongly positively correlated with dependence upon wage work and proportion of men working full-time and most strongly inversely correlated with dependence upon welfare. (Another projection of the biplot not displayed here shows this more clearly.)

These patterns are not likely to be well explained by the age distribution of the population in each district. According to calculations of the absolute number of deaths and average annual age-specific mortality rates from each major cause (table 3.29), circulatory deaths occur most frequently in the age group 60 and above. Indeed, the number is so great that the average annual crude rate of death from this cause would be expected to be highest in the oldest populations. I have said that such elderly populations are found where dependence upon welfare is greatest. But it is not the elderly in the poor districts who die from this cause. Those who die from circulatory disease are found where involvement in the wage economy is greatest, suggesting that wage economy areas are where age-specific rates are the highest. Combined with the field studies of hypertension reported previously, this indicates that there is a relationship between circulatory diseases and increasing involvement in the wage economy.

Regarding deaths from infectious and respiratory diseases (primarily influenza and pneumonia) and symptoms and ill-

TABLE 3.29

DEATHS AMONG NAVAJOS BY CAUSE, 1972–1978

Age	Pop.	Infective and Parasitic #	rate 100,000	Neoplasms #	rate 100,000	Circulatory #	rate 100,000	Respiratory #	rate 100,000	G.I. #	rate 100,000	Symptoms #	rate 100,000	Accidents #	rate 100,000
< 10	32,600	125	54.8	16	7.0	35	15.3	88	38.5	16	7.0	109	47.8	183	80.2
10–19	39,096	7	2.5	7	2.5	13	4.7	9	3.3	4	1.5	18	6.6	328	120.0
20–29	19,751	9	6.5	9	6.5	27	19.5	20	14.5	35	25.3	25	18.1	556	402
30–39	14,233	16	16.0	25	25.0	25	25.0	31	31.1	88	88.3	57	57.2	333	334.1
40–49	10,435	19	26.0	30	41.0	49	67.0	27	36.9	60	82.1	60	82.1	212	290.2
50–59	7,127	18	36.0	52	104.2	88	176.4	29	58.1	48	96.2	46	92.2	137	274.6
> 60	8,914	70	112.2	213	341.3	437	700.3	223	357.4	92	147.4	211	338.2	220	352.6

defined conditions, notice in table 3.29 that they each are responsible for a substantial number of deaths to children below the age of 10 as well as to adults 60 and above. This may account for the weak positive correlation with postneonatal mortality since deaths in infancy and deaths in childhood are likely to be found in the same populations.

The temporal change in patterns of mortality is only incompletely replicated spatially. In the 1970s, crude rates of mortality from man-made, degenerative, and infectious diseases were all positively correlated and highest in areas where dependence upon welfare was lowest and where involvement in the wage economy tended to be highest. Even had I been able to calculate age-adjusted rates, similar patterns would probably have emerged. It is likely that mortality from these different causes truly is higher in wage work populations. The reason is not entirely clear but may be similar to the explanations offered for the increases in mortality and morbidity observed among other populations moving from rural to urban areas. Changes in diet, increased crowding, new situations for which migrants may be inadequately prepared may all contribute to generally higher rates of mortality from all causes. Indeed, this may even be true of the infectious diseases. Cassel (1974) and Dubos (1965) have both noted that as epidemics caused by virulent exogenous microorganisms wane, the infectious diseases that become important are those caused by organisms that are "ubiquitous in the environment, persist in the body without causing obvious harm under ordinary circumstances, and exert pathological effects only when the infected person is under conditions of physiological stress" (Dubos 1965:164–165). Conceivably this is the situation in which the Navajos now find themselves.

As my data are at the aggregate level and in some respects inadequate, it is not fruitful to proceed much beyond these speculations. It may be said, however, that postneonatal mortality rates are highest in the poorest populations; circulatory diseases, followed by gastrointestinal diseases (including cirrhosis of the liver) and accidental deaths, are highest in wage work populations; and infectious diseases (primarily gastroenteritis, influenza, and pneumonia) and symptoms and ill-defined conditions are somewhat ambiguously placed, evidently affecting children in poor populations as well as adults in wage work populations. Having described historical and contemporary patterns of mortality, I turn in the following two chapters to a description of changes in health care beliefs and practices.

Traditional Navajo Health Beliefs and Practices

NAVAJO RELIGION

THROUGHOUT the greater Southwest it has been observed that "in spite of the complex intertwining of ideas, two separate lines of religious practice can . . . be followed out. Oversimplified, they are as follows: The agriculturists tend to develop communal ceremonies, the hunters, personal religious participation" (Underhill 1948:viii). Traditional Navajo religion is an amalgam of these two lines, for the Navajos, originally hunters from the north, mixed with the Pueblos, especially after the rebellion of 1680, and adopted many features of Pueblo religion. Navajo religion is directed toward the maintenance of harmonious relationships between man, nature, and the supernaturals. As illness is a major indicator of disharmony, Navajo religious ritual is predominantly health oriented. This is congruent with the emphasis of hunters upon personal religious participation focused upon the health and well-being of the individual. There are many references to crops in the rituals, "but Navaho ceremonialism does not show the intense preoccupation with maize and its life cycle which characterizes the true farming peoples" (Underhill 1948:x).

It has also been observed that hunters seek visionary experiences and often have shamans whose powers are divinely received rather than acquired through years of apprenticeship. "The pattern of agricultural ceremonies," by contrast, "tends to create standardized ritual with an hereditary officiant, whose power is not the result of a vision but of memorizing a formula, both in words and behavior" (Underhill 1948:viii).

Again Navajo ceremonialism is an amalgam. The most prestigious figure in the hierarchy of religious practitioners is the singer, whose knowledge of a particular ritual is gained over long years of apprenticeship with another practitioner. Below him is the diviner, whose ability to diagnose illness or other troubles is a gift. Upon making a diagnosis, such an individual may refer a patient to a singer, who performs the ceremony appropriate for the diagnosis. In some instances, the Diviner and Singer may be one and the same individual (Reichard 1963). It is reasonable to suppose that the singer is a reflection of the Pueblo influence, whereas the diviner is a lineal descendent of the shaman of the hunter tradition (Luckert 1975).

In many Navajo communities there are also herbalists and bone setters, people with empirical knowledge about more or less effective ways to treat any number of common complaints and symptoms. As shall be discussed in more detail later, Navajos in the past have often equated physicians with herbalists from whom they seek symptomatic relief, while still continuing to have traditional Navajo ceremonies to cure the underlying condition.

It is generally agreed that the number of singers has been declining on the reservation. In a careful study of the Kaibeto Plateau, Henderson (1982:167ff.) reports that there was 1 singer for every 30 people in the area from 1900 through the 1930s. By 1980, however, there was only one for every 175 people. Not only had the population increased from 600 to 4,244 in that time but the number of singers had decreased steadily since the 1950s. Presently the number of practicing singers is about the same as it was at the turn of the century. Of 70 singers who lived in the area between 1860 and 1981, 51 (73 percent) were born before 1900 and only 2 (3 percent) were born after 1930. Moreover, those singers alive today knew fewer ceremonies than did those of earlier years. There is also some evidence that several sings have become extinct and that the ceremonies now performed are increasingly the short one- and three-night versions of longer ceremonies. The reasons for these developments are straightforward: "To learn a chant requires that a man be on the reservation . . . for long periods of time. It also requires leisure and the ability to pay the teacher" (Aberle 1966:201f.). As reliance on wage work increases at the expense of stock raising, it becomes almost impossible for young men to meet these conditions.

Ultimately, education and the demands of the wage work economy will be the nemesis of the traditional healing system. For the present, however, there are several developments that suggest that a period of adaptation and innovation has begun. Since 1970 the Navajo Healing Arts Training Program, funded by the National Institute of Mental Health, has trained some ninety individuals from the central part of the reservation. Because an undetermined number of these trainees were already qualified singers when they entered the program, it is not clear just how many new singers have been trained, nor is it known whether all of these individuals are practicing as full-time healers.

The willingness, under certain circumstances, of the Internal Revenue Service to allow deductions for expenses incurred for Navajo healing ceremonies is another example of changed white attitudes toward traditional medicine. Some Navajos have come to feel that this process of acceptance will be facilitated by the certification of ceremonial practitioners and standardization of fees; thus, in 1979 the Navajo Medicine Men's Association was organized (Shepardson 1982:205f.). Although few singers have agreed to become members, it has become the means by which peyote road chiefs and Navajo hand tremblers and herbalists hope to achieve recognition as bona fide native healers. It is likely that as the number of singers declines, health entrepreneurs such as the hand trembler who has learned some parts of a major healing ceremony may be able to meet the need for an "Indian medicine" to oppose the alien modern system. It is possible that as the traditional system dies, a folk system will take its place, one that will function more as an expression of ethnic independence and pride than as a system of healing or a coherent religion.

During the twentieth century, Christianity and peyotism have gained large followings on the reservation, with implications for changing health concepts and behavior which have not yet been studied. The peyote religion, now formally organized as the Native American Church, is a nativistic religion that began among the Kiowa and Comanche Indians of the south plains during the latter half of the nineteenth century and spread to the tribes of the plains, prairies and Rocky Mountain west. By embracing some central tenets of Christianity in an Indian ritual framework, it provides an Indian answer to the white man's religion. The use of peyote, a small cactus containing several psychoactive alkaloids, notably mescaline, has special appeal to those Indians whose aboriginal religions afforded a prominent position to visions as a means of gaining supernatural power (LaBarre 1938:1960).

Before the stock reduction period of the late 1930s, the Navajos showed little interest in the new religion, although the Utes, their neighbors to the north, had adopted it in the early part of the twentieth century. According to Aberle (1966), the stresses of stock reduction made the Navajos receptive during these years, and he documents the religion's rapid growth in those communities most affected by the reduction program. Peyotism has continued to exert an appeal and to spread across the reservation since that time. In the areas where I have worked, I detect two additional reasons for its continued popularity.

Real income has declined during the past two decades. Regardless of whether this decline has created stress, it has made it more difficult for Navajo families to pay for the large traditional healing ceremonies which last from five to nine nights and involve hosting large numbers of guests. The peyote ceremony lasts only one night and is, consequently, more economical than most Navajo ceremonies. Its ritual is simple, standardized, and not difficult to learn for either the lay participant or the religious leader. As it introduced no new beliefs about the causes of disease and denies none of the central Navajo beliefs, it is easy to use as a substitute for traditional ceremonies. In fact, I have found many families who use both forms of treatment.

The years of apprenticeship necessary to master any of the major Navajo ceremonials make it impossible for young men with wage jobs to achieve status as traditional ceremonialists. The peyote ritual, performed on a single weekend night, is particularly suited to patients and practitioners who must conform to the demands of wage work. Young Navajos who do not have, or want, access to status in the non-Indian world find that becoming a peyote leader gives them status in their own community. As noted above, it is my opinion that economic change has created a shortage of traditional ceremonialists which will become crucial during the next ten years.

The same conditions that have promoted the growth of the Navajo Native American Church have also worked to popularize the fundamentalist Christian denominations. Missionary activities, begun by the Spaniards in the seventeenth century and continued by the more established Protestant denominations after the establishment of the reservation, never gained large numbers of converts before the stock reduction period. The mission church had always been run by non-Indians, thus it was separate from Navajo community life. In recent years, however, the "camp church" has gained popularity because it has Navajo preachers who maintain their place in their kin networks. In 1950, there were 36 organized congregations with pastors, two of whom were Navajo. In 1978, there were 343 congregations, 203 of them with Navajo preachers (DuBois 1978). The greatest growth has been among such groups as the Nazarenes, Pentecostals, and Baptists.

Currently, the Navajo Native American Church claims that 50 percent of the reservation population is peyotist. Comparable figures for the various Christian denominations are not available and all are loose estimates at best. The Mormons, for example, claim that 20,000 Navajos are members of their church, although this count includes individuals who never go to church (*The Navajo Times* 1978:A-2). Where good survey research has been done, all Christian denominations combined comprise from 50 to 70 percent of populations adjacent to new wage work opportunities where skilled workers have migrated into the area. The Navajo Native American Church comprises between 15 and 20 percent of populations in more rural areas, *not* including people who combine peyotism with traditional religion (Callaway et al. 1976:57). These data, however, are from the western portion of the reservation and cannot be generalized to the more densely populated areas to the east where peyotism first took root. The point to be made is that diversity in religious practices is considerable and, while it probably has important consequences for changing health beliefs and behaviors, no research to date has concentrated upon this problem. Without detailed studies that connect religious belief to health behavior, it would be premature to use religious preference as an indicator of changed health behavior. Most stories about the conversion of Navajo adults that I have heard involve the use of Christian prayer or peyote either to cure a specific illness or to protect against witchcraft.

CONCEPTS OF DISEASE AND ILLNESS

According to Navajo belief, disease may be contracted by *soul loss, intrusive object, spirit possession, breach of tabu,* and *witchcraft.* Specific etiologic agents may cause disease by one or more of these means.

The notion of soul loss is not a major means by which specific diseases are caused, yet there is reason to believe that the concept is important to the Navajo. The soul, or wind as it is most often called, enters the body soon after birth and forms the individual's basic personality. At death the soul leaves the body and proceeds to the afterworld. Faintness and suffocation are signs that the wind-soul is leaving the body and signal the final stage of an illness. The child's first laugh indicates that the soul has become attached to the body. Before this, the infant may die easily. During old age once more the soul is loosely attached, and death at this time is considered natural. The ghosts of the very old and of infants are not thought to be potent causes of disease, while those of people who die while the wind-soul is well attached are thought to be potent etiologic agents.

A disease-causing agent, or intrusive object, may be injected into the body by a special form of witchcraft which has been glossed as "wizardry" by Kluckhohn (1962). This form of witchcraft is said to be a recent (nineteenth-century) borrowing from the Pueblos, among whom it is relatively prominent. Neither wizardry nor its cure, the Sucking Way, are central to Navajo healing belief and practices. Sucking Way is said to have been borrowed from the Chiricahua Apaches (Haile 1950). Emaciation, together with pain in that part of the body where the object has lodged, are diagnostic of wizardry.

Spirit intrusion, or possession, involves the displacement of the wind-soul by the spirit of a dangerous being, most often a supernatural. Kaplan and Johnson (1964) maintain that possession is the central concept of disease causation and relate it to what they assert is a predisposition for Navajo mental illnesses to be hysterical in nature. While there are no quantitative data available to either support or deny this assertion, several observations are in order. When Navajos talk about actual cases—how a specific illness was contracted by a particular individual—they never mention spirit intrusion. However, the recorded myths of the healing ceremonies and the ceremonialists with whom I have discussed this matter describe the principal disease in terms of possession. The myth of the Evil Way chant, for example, tells how the supernatural known as Coyote sent his ghost into the hero in order to witch him (Haile 1950). When an individual is possessed by the mythical Gila Monster, that person's arms begin to shake, a sign that he has the gift to diagnose illness by "hand trembling" (Wyman 1936). It is possible that lay people do not know the myths in sufficient detail to be cognizant of the role spirit possession plays. More likely, however, the tendency to avoid implicating spirit possession results from a desire to avoid anxiety-provoking diagnoses. It may be less threatening to hear that one has inadvertently stepped on a coyote track than to learn that one is possessed by Coyote himself.

Breach of tabu includes not only the commission of prohibited acts, such as incest, but also coming into contact with a "dangerous" object. For example, sibling incest is thought to cause generalized seizures. In this instance the breach of a major tabu is involved, and some degree of volition is implied. The Navajos, however, call this disease "moth sickness" and believe that the moth is the principal etiologic agent. The original act of incest was committed by the Butterfly People in the mythical past. Dawn Boy and Dawn Girl, who were watching from the canyon's rim, decided to do the same thing with the result that they too went "wild." They and the Butterfly People became "like moths who fly into the fire," twisting and convulsing. The Moth Way was first performed to cure Dawn Boy and his sister, Dawn Girl (Haile 1937). Moths had lodged themselves behind their eyes and, during the curing ceremony, they spat out moth wings. In effect, they were possessed.

Today, a human with seizures may be diagnosed as suffering from moth sickness because he behaves like a moth. But it is not necessary that actual incest be committed. Utilizing principles of sympathetic magic—like causes have like effects and objects once in contact with each other retain each other's properties—diseases may be contracted through inadvertent contact with an etiologic agent. Thus, moth sickness may also be contracted if a real moth, which shares the properties of the mythical Moth, touches a person. This is also a breach of tabu, although no volition on the part of the individual is involved. Disease-causing objects or beings are considered "dangerous," and the all-embracing rule is: you shall have no contact with anything that is "dangerous." Prenatal influence is included in this class of behaviors. If a pregnant woman breaches a tabu, the child she bears may also contract the illness at a later date. Some form of breach of tabu is the most frequently reported kind of diagnosis. In this context it should also be noted that a witch can make an individual come into contact with a "dangerous" object in order to make him ill. In the example of moth sickness, a witch can either cause the victim to touch a moth or can cause his mind to go "wild" so that the victim will become like a moth. In this event the individual will ultimately commit incest and develop seizures.

Witchcraft is another frequently mentioned means of contracting disease. I have already mentioned that form of witchcraft Kluckhohn has labeled "wizardry." In his monograph on the subject, he mentions three other types: *witchery, sorcery,* and *frenzy witchcraft* (Kluckhohn 1962).

Witchery is the primary form of Navajo witchcraft, and it is mentioned in the creation myth as having been originated by First Man and First Woman. Witches are associated with the dead and with incest, two of the most dangerous etiologic agents. To qualify as a witch an individual must kill a close relative, especially a sibling. In the myths, male witches invariably live in incestuous unions with one of their daughters. Some informants claim that the witch initiate must eat part of a murdered relative's body. The effective means of working witchery is by touching the victim with a powder made from corpse flesh, thus bringing him into contact with a "dangerous" etiologic agent. Most often, witches transform themselves into wolves, coyotes, or dogs but also into bears, owls, foxes, and crows, in order to travel undetected. Witchery mirrors and is the evil opposite of Navajo religion. Not only is it based upon the two great "dangers," incest and death, but witches band together and perform their own ceremonials using chants, sand paintings, body painting, and masks. Informants describe the proceedings as "just like a bad sign" (Kluckhohn 1962:27). As corpse powder is brought into contact with the victim, it is not surprising that the signs of witchery are the same as those of ghost sickness: fainting and unconsciousness.

Sorcery is closely associated with witchery, and sorcerers participate in the witchery ceremonials. Sorcerers use spells to work their evil. The sorcerer must have a bit of the victim's personal excreta (hair, nails, feces, etc.) over which he casts his spell. Even in this instance, however, breach of tabu is involved as the parts of the victim's person are most often buried near a lightning-struck tree, which is "dangerous," or in a grave. Personal excreta or clothing still retain properties of the victim and, because like causes produce like results, what is done to them is also done to the victim.

Frenzy witchcraft is primarily love magic, though it is also used in trading, gambling, and hunting. The master of this form of witchcraft uses a concoction made from datura in much the same way as corpse powder is used in witchery. The datura plant contains scopalomine and hyosciamine and produces hallucinations, dissociative reactions and, in some instances, coma when ingested. According to Navajo belief, the victim has only to be touched by the concoction, although smoking or ingesting it brings about the same results. When women are witched in this manner, they "go out of their minds," run around in circles, sometimes tear off their clothes, and sometimes fall to the ground and lose consciousness. The aim is to make the woman lose her senses and run away from human habitation in a state of sexual frenzy so that the witch can catch and seduce her. When used in gambling against males, the victim goes out of his mind, gambles recklessly, and loses his wealth to the witch.

It is important to remember that witches are believed to be manipulating the etiologic agents that cause the disease. A person said to be witched is thought to have the disease caused by the etiologic agent with which he came into contact, and he should have the ceremony good for that particular agent. Because witchery is so prevalent and because it uses corpse powder, the ceremonial that cures ghost sickness is said to be particularly effective against witchcraft.

Almost anything can cause disease. Even beneficent deities

may be a source of illness if approached improperly. Wyman and Kluckhohn (1938) note that Navajos recognize four classes of etiologic agents: animals, natural phenomena, healing ceremonies, and evil spirits. This discussion will be confined to those etiologies that are the most frequently diagnosed or are considered the most dangerous.

Wyman and Kluckhohn (1938:14) obtained a list of disease-causing animals from an old informant; it included ten mammals, seven reptiles, twelve birds, and all fish. To this should be added at least seven insects (Wyman and Bailey 1964). (In light of the fact that datura can cause illness as well as any plant used for ceremonial purposes, this class might be thought of as including sentient beings of all sorts. It is possible, however, to include the plants with the class of ceremonials as well.) The most frequently invoked beings in this class are the bear, coyote, porcupine, snake, eagle, moth, ant, long-horned grasshopper, and camel cricket. The bear is a powerful and dangerous animal throughout North America and Siberia. Its importance extends back to antiquity and is thought to be central to the Siberian shaman complex that diffused to the New World. Vestiges of a circumpolar paleolithic bear cult have been identified throughout the Arctic (Campbell 1970:339). The coyote is a trickster figure for most of the tribes in the mountain west. He is associated with the central evils of Navajo culture: death, witchcraft, incest, sexual excess, and extreme behavior in general. The deer was a common game animal whose spirit, if offended, would cause illness; diagnoses of deer contamination are becoming less and less common. Snakes and the porcupine are important in Navajo mythology, but why they and the eagle are especially dangerous is open to speculation. The moth, I have already noted, is associated with incest and seizures. Ants are ubiquitous in daily life and are associated with witchcraft. They are often thought to be shot into a victim's body by a wizard. Camel crickets and long-horned grasshoppers are associated with ghosts because they gather around dead bodies. The list is almost endless. Horn worms and darkling beetles, for example, are generally thought to be good but will cause illness if killed.

The most common causes of illness in the class of natural phenomena are lightning and whirlwinds. Water, hail, and the earth itself are mentioned less often. I will venture a naturalistic explanation. Lightning and whirlwinds are common, dramatic, and destructive in a land of sudden, violent summer storms. Lightning is visually generalized to include all things that are long, slender, and move in a zig-zag motion, which thus associates it with arrows and snakes. Lightning is also associated with whirlwinds because storms often display thunder, lightning, and wind at the same time. In Navajo belief there are many kinds of wind, both beneficent and dangerous. Whirlwinds are especially destructive. It is interesting that the two most frequently used healing ceremonials, the Wind and Shooting (lightning) Way chants, not only protect against a broad array of symptoms but also overlap in the domain of causal agents.

Any ceremonial can cause illness. All powerful forces are also dangerous, so that when the Holy People are present during a ceremony an individual may be affected. Individuals who become ill in this way are said to have the same illness the ceremonial is said to cure. Transgressions of tabus—for example, that against cohabitation during a ceremony and for four days afterwards—can cause illness. Breaches of tabus during ceremonies may cause illness in a child through prenatal influence. A common statement of patients is "my mother looked upon a sand painting she was not supposed to see."

In the category of evil spirits, the ghosts of the dead are prominent. The belief that the ghost can affect the living deleteriously is a common and, probably, ancient belief among North American Indians. The Navajos believe that any contact with the corpse, the house where death has occurred, places once occupied by the ancients (i.e., the Pueblo ruins), and even old artifacts will cause ghost sickness. A variety of mythical monsters are also included in this class, although diagnoses involving them are rare at present.

In the opinion of most observers, Navajos classify disease by etiologic agent, and each healing ceremony is known by the causal factors it is thought to cure. At the same time, however, there appear to be some operational classifications somewhat apart from the explicit formalization of Navajo disease theory. I have already mentioned the concern for a variety of behavioral symptoms labeled as "excess frenzy" or "going to extremes." These behaviors include insanity, dissociative states, and convulsions, among others, and tend to be associated with some of the more "dangerous" etiologic agents such as bear, coyote, moth, and ghosts. The tabus against incest and witchcraft are also associated with these etiologies. There is, in my opinion, some possibility that the Navajos assign a special importance to symptoms we generally associate with mental disorders. Navajos also recognize that some diseases are contagious, or "going around," though this may be a postcontact development, as there are no etiologies specifically said to cause such maladies. Distinctions made between white and Navajo diseases have been noted in the literature and will be discussed below.

Despite the fact that Navajos make use of modern medicine, as well as of curers from neighboring tribes, peyote ceremonies, Christian ministers and, upon occasion, faith healers, there has been remarkably little incorporation of these foreign ideas into the traditional belief system. This is due, I believe, to two things: (1) the healing system is sacred, the very core of Navajo religion, and (2) healing ceremonies aim to remove the cause of disease and do not directly attempt to alleviate symptoms, thus leaving the patient free to seek relief by any means available to him. In consequence, I feel justified in discussing the traditional belief system without considering influences other systems may exert upon it. Utilization of other medical systems does not necessarily imply a corresponding change in concepts on the part of the patient. Individuals, however, do change, and the extent to which health beliefs have and are changing is an area that must be investigated empirically.

Because Navajo religion is remarkably complex, it is not surprising to find considerable differences in medical knowledge between the young and the old and between the layman and the professional. The typical traditional Navajo learns from childhood which tabus must be observed to avoid illness. Exactly how these tabus derive from the myths of the healing ceremonies, however, is not always well understood by the layman. I found repeatedly that many Navajo patients did not know why a ceremonial was performed for them, beyond the fact that the diagnostician had recommended it. Some families had more medical knowledge than did others, often because of the presence of a ceremonialist in the extended family. As a rule, children of ceremonialists knew more about traditional medical concepts than other children.

Learning a major ceremonial can take as long as eight years of apprenticeship. Most ceremonialists specialize in only one or two complete ceremonies and know the short forms of several others. The shift to a wage work economy has made it almost impossible for most young men to find the time to learn the ceremonials. To date, increased transportation and a growing network of paved roads have permitted ceremonialists to serve a larger number of patients. It is possible, however, that there will be an acute shortage of knowledgeable ceremonialists in another ten years.

Virtually all Navajo children attend school and are exposed to some basic modern ideas of disease causation. In addition, Navajos come into contact with whites in a variety of contexts. Health information is disseminated by the Indian Health Service, and increasing numbers of Navajos are choosing careers in the health professions. There is no doubt that the general level of understanding is improving.

To date there are no published studies assessing the extent to which different segments of the Navajo population understand modern health concepts. Nor is there adequate information about differences in health concepts attributable to adherence to Christianity or peyotism. While each religion claims that faith can cure, and the peyotists believe that the peyote plant is a great medicine, it is not known whether either religion has formulated its own distinct notions about disease causation or classification.

It is important to note that the traditional healing system persists with remarkable internal consistency across a reservation the size of West Virginia and that the ceremonies and normative beliefs are practically identical with those documented at the turn of the century. Individuals may cease to believe in the old ways, but to date there is little evidence to suggest that Navajo traditional beliefs have incorporated new concepts or curing techniques. Adair and Deuschle quote a prominent politician and ceremonialist as saying that there are diseases (a) that the Navajos cannot cure but that White physicians can; (b) that both physicians and ceremonialists can cure; and (c) that only Navajo ceremonialists can cure (Adair and Deuschle 1970:33). In my opinion, it would be erroneous to infer from this public statement that Navajo ceremonialists currently have a new category called "white diseases" which they recognize and for which they recommend modern therapy. The example most often mentioned in this regard is tuberculosis, which the Navajos have learned can be cured by antibiotic therapy. Tuberculosis, however, is not diagnosable by Navajo methods, and I have never encountered a patient who was diagnosed as having either a white disease or tuberculosis. What I do observe is a growing acceptance of modern medicine based upon its demonstrated effectiveness. Neither ceremonialists nor their patients are averse to seeking treatment from physicians. It has not always been so, however. Prior to the introduction of antibiotics and therapy for tuberculosis, modern medicine did not cure an impressive number of tuberculosis or pneumonia patients. In fact, before the 1950s, tubercular patients faced incarceration in a sanatoria without certain recovery. The Navajos looked upon hospitals and sanatoria as houses of death where it was almost certain the patient would contract ghost sickness. Navajo acceptance of the hospital has changed as the rate of cure has improved, so that today a ceremonialist may tell a patient to do what the white doctors say rather than telling him to stay away at all costs. The change in attitude, however, does not imply a change in the traditional system itself.

Though differences among peyotism, traditional Navajo religion, and Navajo Christianity do exist, it is doubtful that these differences reflect corresponding differences in health concepts. Traditionalists and peyotists share a belief in witchcraft as a cause of disease. So, too, do Navajo Christians, with the exception of the more acculturated and educated. Indeed, several informants report that they became Christians because it was a strong protection against witchcraft. Others say they could no longer afford ceremonials so they tried Christianity because they heard that Jesus was stronger than any witch and could cure any disease. Recently, a Christian Navajo preacher described how the peyotists in his community had tried to witch his entire congregation and how he had waged a twenty-four-hour battle against the spell that caused the congregation to scream and lose consciousness. Acculturation and education are better predictors of changed health concepts than is religious affiliation per se. At the same time, however, it must be pointed out that the more educated Navajos tend to be Christian, peyotist, or unaffiliated. Finally, although peyotists and Christians do not utilize Navajo healing ceremonies, the traditionalist is likely to attend peyote ceremonies upon occasion and may even consider himself a member of both religions. Traditionalists will also attend church gatherings, and virtually all Navajos utilize modern medicine.

BECOMING ILL

Navajos tend to classify diseases by cause rather than by symptom. In consequence it is difficult to determine precisely the role symptoms play in diagnosis. No Navajo disease is known by the symptoms it produces or by the part of the body it is thought to affect. Rather, there is bear sickness and porcupine sickness, named for the agents thought to cause them; or there is "that which is treated by the Shooting Chant," so named by the ceremonials used to cure it. Because the traditional health culture does not rely upon a knowledge of symptoms in the diagnostic process, Navajo patients often have difficulty understanding the purpose of history taking and physical examination, a circumstance that often leads to misunderstanding in the clinical setting.

Despite the foregoing, however, Navajos do recognize that they are ill by the discomfort they experience, and some symptoms appear to have special meaning for them. There is no reason to believe, as many physicians have suggested, that Navajos are poor observers (Leighton and Kennedy 1957). Landar (1967) has shown that the language of pain among Navajos is sophisticated, and it is my experience that their symptoms are well described and that Navajos are good historians when it is made clear to them why a physician needs to have a good history of their condition.

Wyman and Kluckhohn (1938) have noted a loose association both between etiological agents and disease categories and between etiologic agents and symptoms. A single cause may produce any of several symptoms and, conversely, a single symptom may be caused by any of several etiologic agents. Several diagnoses and treatments may be tried before the correct one is determined. Nevertheless, certain groups of healing ceremonies appear to be associated with some symptoms and not others, while several other ceremonies appear to be good for a broad range of symptoms. The Evil Way chants, Moth Way, Hand Trembling Way, the Mountain Way chant group, and, perhaps, Coyote Way appear to be associated with behavioral symptoms regardless of whether these symptoms are organic or functional in origin. One may tentatively infer from this a distinction between what may be called "mental" disorders and all others. Similarly, the ceremonies in which supernaturals are impersonated (Night Way and Plume Way) are thought to be good primarily for head problems, especially deafness and blindness, while other ceremonies, especially the Shooting Way chants, are said to be effective for a large variety of common disorders sucn as colds, fevers, abdominal pain, joint pain and swelling, muscle soreness, and the like. The fact that the Shooting Way and Wind Way chants are among the most frequent ceremonies may be due largely to their reputations as cures for a wide range of symptoms.

The question remains whether patients are diagnosed and treated according to their actual symptoms or whether more random, magical considerations come into play. For, while informants believe that certain ceremonies are good for certain symptoms, they also maintain that a given ceremony will be used to cure a disease caused by a specific etiologic agent regardless of the symptoms. Thus, the Shooting Way may be considered especially good for bodily aches and pains, but it will also be used for insanity if the latter is diagnosed as being caused by lightning or snakes, the etiologic agents this chant is especially aimed at. Remarkably little quantitative research has been done correlating reported symptoms with native diagnoses and treatments for any sizable number of patients.

One study has attempted to determine the degree to which Navajos distinguish various types of epileptic seizures one from another, whether epileptic seizures are distinguished from hysterical seizures (conversion reactions), and whether seizure patients actually receive the native diagnoses and treatments Navajo informants claim are especially effective in curing these symptoms (Levy et al. 1977; Levy, in press; Neutra et al. 1977). Navajo tradition gives a prominent position to (a) the signs of grand mal seizure, said to be caused by sibling incest; (b) the signs of psychomotor seizure or any bout of irrational behavior that culminates with the patient falling to the ground and losing consciousness, attributed to a form of witchcraft; (c) unilateral convulsions, shaking or trembling, thought to indicate the gift of "hand trembling," the major method of diagnosing disease. Adequate data were gathered from 11 epileptics, 7 of whom had conversion reactions in addition to their epileptic convulsions, and from 9 patients with conversion reactions that looked like seizures. (In addition, 5 traditional epileptics and 1 "hysteric" had had no ceremonies performed for them, while 3 epileptics and 1 "hysteric" were acculturated and relied only upon nontraditional forms of treatment.) The ceremonies performed for the 20 individuals who utilized Navajo ceremonial treatments were documented from the time of onset to the time of the initial interview. The profile of ceremonies obtained was then compared with the ceremonies performed for two groups of Navajos, one rural and the other living near a government settlement, over a five-year period. This control group of 208 individuals of all ages displayed a broad array of typical health problems ranging from upper respiratory tract infections and gastrointestinal problems to gallbladder disease. None of them had seizures or suffered from any behavioral disorders.

Seizure patients and controls alike utilized such ceremonies as the Shooting Way and the Wind Way, thought to be good for a wide variety of symptoms. Both groups used the Evil Way chant with some frequency, a ceremony thought to be effective for fainting and anxiety attacks but not for seizures or insanity. Over 90 percent of all ceremonies performed for the control group patients were in this class of popular ceremony, while only 60 percent of all ceremonies performed for the seizure patients were in this category. Both groups used the Night Way and the Plume Way ceremonies, which are expensive, and the rare Earth and Beauty Ways; these ceremonies constituted from 5 to 6 percent of the total for both groups. While these are not thought to be good for seizures, they are especially noted for their effectiveness against head ailment, abdominal pains, and joint inflammation and swelling. Both controls and seizure patients used Life Way and Flint Way, which are for injuries and chronic disorders of all sorts (seizure patients, 4 percent; controls, 2 percent). Importantly, no ceremonies thought to be good specifically for seizurelike behavior (Coyote Way, Hand Trembling Way, Frenzy Witchcraft Way, Moth Way, Mountain Top Way, and various minor ceremonies such as the Twirling Basket ritual) were utilized by the control group, while 30 percent of all ceremonies performed for the seizure patients were of this type. The differences between the two groups in terms of their use of healing ceremonies were significant and led to the conclusion that symptoms and signs are of some importance in determining the appropriate treatments, at least in the domain investigated.

The chronicity of symptoms is an important factor in the process of diagnosing and classifying disease. In the above-mentioned study, 9 of 11 epileptics with grand mal seizures who had ceremonial treatment ultimately used ceremonies said to be good especially for generalized seizures. None of the 3 patients with conversion reactions that emulate generalized seizures had these sings performed for them. The difference between the two groups was significant ($p = .03$ by Fisher's Exact Test). The epileptic patients, regardless of seizure type, received the treatments appropriate for their seizures significantly more often than did the hysterical patients ($p = .01$ by Fisher's Exact Test). I do not think these differences are due to an ability to accurately distinguish between an epileptic seizure and a conversion reaction but to the fact that epileptic seizures persisted for years while the conversion reactions were more transient. Seizure-specific ceremonies were only resorted to after a number of other ceremonies had been tried, even though some epileptics were diagnosed as needing such a ceremony soon after the onset of their seizures. It is not known whether less startling signs and symptoms than those of epilepsy are used to determine the diagnosis or the treatment of other disorders with sufficient frequency to offset the tendency to try several treatments and so produce statistically significant associations between symptoms and treatments.

There have been virtually no organized investigations of Navajo tolerance for pain or for different symptoms. Over the years, the clinical experience of numerous physicians indicates that, in general, Navajos tend to regard themselves as sick according to the degree of pain they experience rather than by the appearance of symptoms per se. In addition, Navajos appear more stoical than white patients (Leighton and Kennedy 1957). In my opinion, however, there is no evidence to suggest that the threshold of pain is higher among Navajos, although this has been suggested by some physicians working on the reservation. It seems more likely that poor people who lead harsh lives find that seeking treatment is costly and should not be undertaken casually. Thus, Navajos tend to put up with ailments that cause little discomfort and do not impair function. In consequence, while the presence of disease may be recognized, treatment may not be sought until the pain is great and the individual cannot function adequately. Prior to this, most Navajos tend not to talk about their pain to the family in order not to worry them. Navajos living close to a hospital and thus avoiding transportation costs tend to use the physician more frequently.

There is some reason to believe that mental disorders are of special concern to Navajos. "Mind loss" manifested by faints, dissociative reactions, and seizures are thought to be the final stage of most, if not all, diseases. In fact, many Navajo informants have said that they recognized they were ill when they experienced anxiety-provoking dreams that had no obvious cause. Whether there is less tolerance for such symptoms—in the sense that treatment will be sought sooner when these symptoms occur or will provoke more anxiety than would be occasioned by other symptoms—is a moot question.

Extremes of behavior, especially violence, appear to signal the need for treatment (Kaplan and Johnson 1964). In 1962 and 1963, Levy interviewed most of the schizophrenic patients seen in the Tuba City Hospital ($n=16$). Despite the facts that these patients did not exhibit overt violence and that few were diagnosed as paranoid, the admission records of the male patients did contain accounts of violence. During the interview, however, patients and families maintained that actual violence had not taken place but that treatment had been sought because they feared it might if something were not done to avert it. Patients would say something like, "I was afraid I might hurt my wife and children." It seems that a potential for violence signals the need for treatment more effectively than other, more typical symptoms of schizophrenia do. In contrast to the male schizophrenic, females were brought to the hospital after they had become so withdrawn that they could no longer cook for their families or, as was sometimes mentioned, weave. Hallucinations, delusions, and disorientation were rarely the symptoms described by families at time of admission.

A number of congenital malformations, such as cleft palate, appear to be negatively labeled by the community. Others, such as supernumerary digits and congenital hip displacement, excite no comment (Adair and Deuschle 1970). The high prevalence of these latter disorders probably accounts for their greater acceptance. Twin births are disvalued and are thought to be caused by promiscuity as well as by chance. The survival rate of twins has been shown to be poor, even taking into account the tendency for twins to be born prematurely (Levy 1964a). The hermaphrodite, by contrast, has occupied a valued position (Hill 1935), at least until recently.

Because of the belief that generalized seizures are caused by sibling incest, many epileptic patients lead difficult lives. Female epileptics, for example, have had records of incest, promiscuity, illegitimate births, and heavy drinking significantly more often than have hysterical females with conversion reactions that look like seizures ($p = .01$ by Fisher's Exact Test). Even considering incest, rape, and illegitimate births separately, the difference is still significant ($p = .04$): none of the 10 female "hysterics" had these problems, while 4 of the 10 female epileptics did. In fact, 3 of the epileptics in the Tuba City Service Unit had actually committed sibling incest. After the onset of seizures, the female loses her value as a potential mate and is open to exploitation by male relatives. These cases occurred in less wealthy and somewhat disorganized families. By contrast, more wealthy, traditional families reared their epileptic children in isolation to protect them from community censure, and these children did not have problems of the sort described. Ten of the 11 male epileptics for whom there was adequate information had problems with alcohol. Four of these were prone to violence, and one had committed sibling incest. Because drinking is prevalent among Navajo males generally and because there was only 1 male "hysteric" in the study, it is not certain whether these problems are more prevalent among male epileptics than among the general Navajo population.

The seizure patients in the Tuba City Service Unit sample were followed for a period of eleven years (1964–1974). During this period, 4 of the 11 epileptics died from unknown or unnatural causes (suspected suicide, 1; exposure after drinking, 2; cause undetermined, 1). All but the suspected suicide were females. It is my impression that these deaths are unusual even for epileptics, but I have no hard data for comparative purposes from other cohorts of epileptics in other populations. Only one "hysteric" died during this period, and this was from old age. The only epileptics who avoided social problems were those reared in isolation and the very acculturated who were well maintained on medication.

No research has been done on how Navajos discuss their symptoms within the family, larger kin group, or community. Although we know that families sometimes make a diagnosis without consulting a diagnostician, the very fact that traditional methods of diagnosis do not utilize symptoms indicates that such discussions may not be a routine matter. Before being diagnosed, Navajos have a number of expressions they use to indicate the degree of discomfort they feel (Werner 1965; Levy 1964b; Leighton and Kennedy 1957). Werner and Levy maintain that these expressions, though using terms for aches and fever, do not imply the presence of any specific type of pain. Leighton and Kennedy, by contrast, feel that "feeling bad all over" indicates the presence of one of a small number of disease syndromes which the authors do not identify. My guess is that, most often, an individual will express the degree of pain experienced rather than the specific symptoms, unless there is obvious trauma such as a broken leg.

Nevertheless, Navajos do discuss observable signs, as the data from the epilepsy study suggest. It is also reasonable to assume that, in matrifocal households, daughters feel free to discuss their own and their childrens' symptoms with their mothers and maternal aunts. While it is known that problems of patient management are discussed in the family setting, it is unclear whether symptoms are discussed in the same way. Husbands and wives are often reticent to discuss health matters with each other when they involve "women's problems." Kunitz (1976b) has found that there was remarkably little communication between female kinsmen concerning birth control and female sexuality. In sum, though Navajos learn about disease and though symptoms do not go completely undiscussed, patterns of communication are not known to outside investigators.

When comparing the role symptoms play in the process of seeking help among the Navajos with what has been reported for the poor in general (McKinlay 1975), one finds similarities owing to poverty and differences owing to culture. The poor in general react to pain rather than to any specific symptom, as do the

Navajo. Economic considerations tend to make health concerns take low priority. At the same time, however, the Navajos appear to be sensitive to such symptoms as violence and irrationality in the same way that various ethnic groups in the general population seem to react more quickly to some symptoms rather than to others.

The discussion thus far has dealt exclusively with traditional Navajo patients. Yet between 20 and 37 percent of male household heads and higher proportions of their spouses were found to be Christian in areas surveyed by the Lake Powell Research Project, while between 4 and 18 percent were peyotists (Callaway et al. 1976). In addition, the population is more educated now than it has ever been. While it is important to know how acculturation affects health behavior, there are no field studies that have actually compared traditional with nontraditional Navajos. On the behavioral level, however, some obvious general statements may be made. Christians, more educated Navajos, and those reared away from the reservation as a rule do not use traditional Navajo healing ceremonies. None of the patients of this type in the epilepsy study were obtained by the Lake Powell Research Project (unpublished data), and what changes have occurred in the perception of symptoms among these groups is not known.

Peyotists fall into two groups: those who claim to be peyotists only, and those who claim adherence to both peyotist and traditionalist religions. My impression is that definitions of disease and symptom perception are not radically different between peyotists and traditionalists if level of education is controlled for. Peyotists, however, rely upon peyote leaders both for diagnosis and for treatment, despite the fact that the cause and understanding of the malady is often expressed in traditional terms.

COPING WITH ILLNESS OUTSIDE THE MAINSTREAM MEDICAL SYSTEM

Mothers are responsible for the care of their infants and young children; both parents are responsible for their minor children in general. Adults are responsible for the care of their aged parents, and close kinsmen are relied upon to help implement decisions by providing economic support. Although these general statements sound much like the role responsibilities of the white American middle class, there are some important differences. The most obvious one is the degree of autonomy given to individuals, even to relatively young children. White health workers are often nonplused when, after asking whether a child is following a prescribed course of treatment, for example, the mothers says, "Why don't you ask him?" A field health nurse once asked Levy what she ought to do in a case that involved an eleven-year-old boy with an incurable condition who would not take his medication and whose mother insisted it was the boy's choice. After following advice to talk directly with the boy, the nurse was surprised to find that he had an adequate understanding of his illness and that his decision not to take medication was a reasonable and intelligent one. According to the patient, he had decided to discontinue medication and to face almost certain death because continuing to come to the hospital and being restricted in his activities worked considerable hardship on his mother and, in effect, took food out of the mouths of his brothers and sisters. It pained him to see his mother neglect his younger siblings because of her concern for him, and he felt that as there was no hope for a cure in any case, it was best for all concerned that the family return to a normal state as soon as possible.

Physicians and nurses have often commented on the fact that parents seem remarkably unaware of their children's symptoms and appear uncaring and callous. I do not think this is due to a conscious extension of the idea that it is up to each individual to decide when he is ill or to any lack of concern and affection for the children. Rather, I think it has something to do with the already discussed tendency for poor people living in harsh conditions to react only to the most obvious signs in others and to considerable pain of their own. I have had occasion to discuss this with a few articulate women, all of whom said that they just do not react and sometimes hardly notice running noses, coughs, fevers, diarrhea, and loss of appetite. They only become concerned when the child can hardly move. This despite the fact that they are good observers of their own symptoms. It is also quite clear that this pattern is changing as more and more mothers are educated and have more contact with whites.

There are many plants thought to be good home treatments for a large variety of symptoms. Navajos who have a knowledge of these plants and who are able to obtain them will utilize them much as the general population uses aspirin, Kaopectate, or any other popular across-the-counter remedy. Many of these plants have been identified (Elmore 1944; Wyman and Harris 1951), but little work has been done on their actual effectiveness. Elmore has identified thirty-seven plants applied externally and another sixty-two that are ingested (Elmore 1944:96, 97). It is my impression that across-the-counter remedies, readily available at trading posts and at cash-and-carry stores, are rapidly superceding the old herbal remedies.

In the old days, many Navajos had mastered the art of setting bones and cauterizing wounds. Currently, patients with these conditions are almost invariably brought to a hospital or clinic. Heat treatment was and still is used for aches, pains, swelling, and broken bones. The affected part is placed over a pit of hot coals and covered with blankets. This form of treatment is being superceded by modern medical practices, however. The sweat bath remains popular as a home treatment for a large variety of symptoms. It is also the primary means of bathing where there is no running water and is of ceremonial importance as a means of ritual purification. Emetics are used during ceremonies but not as home remedies unless a family member is a ceremonialist or herbalist. I have not detected any pattern of preferring to treat some symptoms as home but not others. Nor is there enough knowledge about the prevalence of home treatments, their benefits or their dangers, for any general statements to be made at this time.

The issue of release from role responsibility is another area where our knowledge is deficient. My impression is that the autonomy allowed each individual in deciding when he is ill and when he needs treatment permits him to withdraw from his role responsibilities before diagnosis and treatment. I have already mentioned, however, that the cessation of functions is, itself, a sign of the need for treatment and that most individuals tend to continue their routine activities until discomfort is quite severe.

The physician's recommendation that a patient be cared for at home and remain relatively inactive places a considerable burden on the family. Initially, resources are mobilized to care for the invalid. Children may be kept home from school to help out, and efforts are made to obtain transportation so that the patient can return to the hospital for follow-up treatments. If the condition does not improve, however, family resources dwindle, and the education of the child kept home from school suffers. At this point, the family is likely to ask that the patient be kept in hospital. Frequently, especially when the patient is elderly or an infant, the family may slacken its efforts. All too often these behaviors are interpreted by physicans as evidence of indifference or irresponsibility.

Another topic about which little is known is lay consultation and referral. While there is no doubt that considerable discussion about health problems takes place within the nuclear and extended family and, frequently, within the wider kin network, actual patterns of consultation have not been accurately ascertained. One study, however, conducted in the 1960s (Levy 1962*b*), does provide some information about the kinds of symptoms for which native ceremonies were used as compared with those for which modern treatments were sought.

Over a two-year period, 77 decisions were made either to seek or not to seek treatment for symptoms recognized by the patient (or a responsible adult in the case of minor children) as indicating the presence of illness in a group of kinsmen comprising 106 individuals of all ages who lived some twenty miles from an Indian Health Service Hospital. Of the 77 instances of recognized illness, only 10 resulted in a decision *not* to seek treatment outside the home. This remarkably high proportion (87%) of decisions to seek medical help from professionals, whether native practitioners or physicians, may be an artifact of the research design, which allowed individuals to define the point at which illness occurred rather than asking about the appearance of symptoms.

Five of the 10 decisions not to seek treatment were made by mothers for infants or young children. There was 1 case of general malaise (later diagnosed as a mild iron deficiency after Levy took the child to the hospital), 2 cases of upper respiratory infection, and 2 cases of measles. Measles had broken out in one family, and the older sibling (aged 13) had been taken to the hospital. The younger children, aged 3 and 4, had not been seen by a physician because their mother did not believe their symptoms were as acute as those of the older brother.

One instance of upper respiratory infection of an adult went untreated. Two cases of adults with diarrhea were treated with unidentifiable pills obtained from a trading post. An adult with vague pains decided against treatment, and an elderly, asymptomatic woman who knew she had come into contact with lightning and needed a ceremonial was overruled by her granddaughter who was the head of the extended family and who felt the family did not have the resources to contract for a five-night ceremonial.

As a general rule, adults defined when they were ill and needed treatment and were also able to decide which form of treatment they required. Adult heads of extended families had the final decision when large outlays of money were involved.

Earlier I mentioned that Navajos tend to use both native and modern therapies for the same illness because of the belief that modern medicine removes symptoms while Navajo medicine cures the illness itself. Although there are no detailed studies of Christians and peyotists, it is my impression that Christians will use modern medicine while using prayer to help obtain a cure, whereas the peyotists are more like the traditionalists in the way they combine or select one form of treatment over another. The study of decisions to seek treatment already discussed (Levy 1962*b*) serves as a convenient starting point for the discussion.

After excluding decisions not to seek treatment, there were 67 instances involving an initial choice to seek either native or modern forms of treatment. In 32 instances (48%) only modern medical care was utilized. Twenty-six decisions (39%) involved utilizing both native healers and physicians, while only 9 (13%) involved the exclusive use of native practitioners. Modern treatment was utilized for fractures, lacerations, and childbirth significantly more often than for all other problems combined (table 4.1). Faints, vague symptoms, and culturally defined illnesses without symptoms were never treated by physicians alone. From this I infer that bodily injuries from accidents, along with childbirth, tend to be viewed as "natural" occurrences which do not, of themselves, require ceremonial cure. Physicians appear to have supplanted herbalists in the population studied.

In addition to the Navajo ceremonialist, native healers from neighboring tribes are sometimes sought. The people in our sample lived within easy driving distance of several Hopi Indian villages. The Hopi are believed to be powerful witches who utilize the method of shooting an object into a victim, and Hopi

TABLE 4.1

USE OF PHYSICIANS AND NATIVE PRACTITIONERS FOR SELF-DEFINED
ILLNESS AMONG 106 INDIVIDUALS OVER A TWO-YEAR PERIOD

Symptoms and conditions	Physician only	Both	Native only
Childbirth and trauma[1]	23	7	0
All others[2]	9	19	9

$X^2 = 19.6$; $d.f. = 2$; $p = .001$

[1]Childbirth; prenatal and postnatal complications and examinations; fractures, lacerations, contusions.

[2]Problems of respiratory systems, including tuberculosis, pneumonia and upper respiratory infections; muscle and joint pain, including arthritis; deafness; crippling, including congenital hip displacement; blindness (cataracts); rashes, sores, and abcesses, including impetigo; diarrhea; faints; conditions ultimately diagnosed as diabetes, prostate infection, thrombosis, urinary tract infection, measles, and chicken pox; vague complaints and malaise; "lightning contamination" (no symptoms) and nightmares.

healers are thought to be experts at curing this as well as other forms of witchcraft. Of 35 instances in which native healers were used, 5 involved the exclusive use of Hopi practitioners. In 1 case, Hopi and Navajo treatments were used jointly, and in another, Hopi treatment was combined with a visit to the hospital. Hopi treatments, in the cases documented as well as in those observed by Levy performed for Hopi patients, were what is known as "sucking" cures. They involve, in addition to "seeing" the cause of the illness, the process of "sucking" the intrusive object from the patient's body. Navajo patients have come from as far away as Shiprock to seek help from Hopi practitioners, despite the fact that Ute sucking shamans are used extensively in the northeastern part of the reservation.

Since the 1960s when this study was conducted, the activities of peyotist and fundamentalist Christian missionaries have increased greatly in the area occupied by the study population. Between 1956 and 1960, no peyote ceremonies were performed for individuals in the population studied. Between 1961 and 1965, although the number of native treatments for the group remained the same, 78 percent were peyote ceremonies. Economic factors and the growing shortage of qualified ceremonialists are the major reasons for this increased reliance on peyote ritual cures (Levy and Kunitz 1974:129). At the height of this religion's popularity, about 28 percent of all adults in the area under consideration claimed membership in the Navajo Native American Church (peyotist), another 25 percent claimed to be adherents to traditional Navajo religion only, and 21 percent were Christian. During the 1970s, interest in peyotism waned somewhat. Traditional Navajo religion continued its decline, and Christianity became more popular (peyotist only, 17%; traditional and peyote, 21%; traditional only, 14%; Christian, 38% [Callaway et al. 1976:57]). The point to be made is that the use of alternative ceremonial treatments varies from community to community and, within a community, over time.

In a survey of hospital use in two populations conducted in the early 1960s (Levy 1962a), it was found that the major variable influencing the frequency of hospital use was distance from the hospital. The closer a population lived to the hospital, the greater the frequency of use. These findings have been replicated by research conducted in the 1970s by the Navajo Health Authority (May et al. 1977; Stewart et al. 1980). By 1965, there were no individuals in the populations studied who never used modern medicine.

To date there are insufficient data to determine whether ceremonial cures have either a beneficial or deleterious effect on any specific diseases. The Navajo predilection for using modern and traditional therapy conjointly indicates that poor utilization of services is less the result of adherence to native beliefs than of difficulties of access to hospitals and of poor communication between patients and medical staffs.

5

Health Care Utilization

THROUGHOUT the first half of the nineteenth century, the administration of Indian affairs was under the jurisdiction of the War Department. From time to time military physicians treated Indian patients, including giving smallpox vaccinations. In 1849 when Indian affairs were transferred to the Department of the Interior, civilian physicians were recruited, and within twenty-five years about half the reservations had a physician.

Services increased slowly in the late nineteenth and early twentieth centuries. Small hospitals were first opened on the Navajo reservation around 1900. From 58 hospital beds in 1912, the number increased to 184 in 1920. This does not include mission hospitals or the 35-bed Hopi hospital at Keams Canyon (established in 1916), which also treated Navajos. The number of admissions fluctuated yearly but generally increased: from 214 in 1912 to 1,092 (including the Hopi hospital) in 1920 (Commissioner of Indian Affairs 1912–1920).

The facilities themselves as well as the quality of medical care provided were regarded by most observers as sadly deficient. In her reminiscences of a tour of Indian Office hospitals on the Navajo reservation in the mid-1920s, Gregg (1965:104) described some of them as "shabby and derelict" and "rattle trap." And while some of the staff were dedicated and competent, others were described as "no-account" and "stupid." Similar observations were made, though more diplomatically, in the Meriam (1928) Report. Care was almost entirely curative, little in the way of prevention being attempted; supplies were inadequate; vital statistics were scarcely collected; and staff were undertrained, isolated, and poorly compensated.

By the early 1930s, bed capacity of hospitals serving the Navajos was 352. Occupancy rates varied considerably but in general were high, often exceeding 100 percent (see table 5.1). Commenting on his experience as a physician on the Navajo Reservation in 1932–1933, Tillim (1936:391) wrote:

The medical work consists of three distinct types of services: the hospitalized cases; the hospital clinic; field dispensing. It is a well-

TABLE 5.1
NAVAJO HOSPITALS, 1933

| Facility | Established | Rated capacity* | | | Average occupancy | |
		Beds	Cribs	Bassinets	#	%
Fort Defiance Sanatorium	1916	28	–	–	27	96.4
Southern Navajo General Hospital	1930	77	3	4	70	83.3
Chinle Hospital	1929	12	–	1	16	123.0
Tohatchi Hospital	1929	10	1	3	16	114.3
Kayenta Sanatorium	1929	52	4	–	43	76.8
Leupp Hospital	1927	28	1	1	29	96.7
Western Navajo Hospital	1928	29	1	1	35	112.9
Winslow Sanatorium	1934	45	–	–	not open	–
Charles Burke Hospital (school infirmary)	1927	34	1	4	16	41.0
Eastern Navajo Hospital	1915	24	2	4	25	83.3
Northern Navajo Hospital	1912	44	–	2	52	113.0
Toadlena Hospital	1929	14	–	2	12	85.7
Total		352			393	111.0

Source: Mountin and Townsend 1936

*Capacity is computed on the basis of 80 square feet per bed unless ceiling height is less than 9 feet, in which case 720 cubic feet per bed is allowed.

established practice to admit for hospitalization any Indian running a temperature and willing to accept treatment. The diagnostic facilities in the hospitals are most inadequate; only two hospitals have x-ray machines. The smaller hospitals have only makeshift provisions for routine blood and urine examination. At times during the school year the hospitals are so overcrowded as to require placing more than one patient in a bed. The Indians' mode of living and lack of intelligence in things medical, make it necessary to hospitalize more often than in a civilized community since home care is a risky undertaking. The hospital clinic is, in reality, a dispensary. Many come for simple remedies for relatives at home.

The New Deal brought major changes in the administration of Indian affairs, including health care. The bureaucracy expanded in size, and the Washington office assumed an increasingly administrative rather than merely advisory role (Gregg 1965:148). In addition, the "anthropological approach" was introduced, though it was viewed with much skepticism by veterans of the Indian service as the largely irrelevant ideas of reformers who accompanied John Collier into office when he was appointed Commissioner of Indian Affairs (Gregg 1965: 142; Philp 1977:166; Kunitz 1971).

Collier's vision of Indian life had considerable impact upon his notions of the importance of clinical medicine. In an address to state and provincial health officers in 1933, he pointed out that the Indian population had increased in some places and declined in others without any relationship to the availability of medical services.

> Now it must be apparent from what I have said that evidently something else than mere clinical services has been a determining factor in the rise and fall of Indian populations heretofore, inasmuch as we see populations rising with no clinical service, and falling where they have them; that there must be something else, important as the clinical services are.
>
> That is the environment, we will just say, in a broad way, which means everything and nothing, that the rise and fall of Indian populations is an expression of the economic and social environment which the Indian has, and that environment for the majority of the Indians now is predominantly white, irrevocably white, and

that is the condition, no matter what we say about it, and no matter now or hereafter what we may try to do about it. (Collier 1933:59)

He went on to point out that the California Indians and various Sioux tribes had been dispossessed and were in decline, whereas Southwestern tribes who still maintained their land base had not declined and in some instances had increased in number. He concluded:

I do not myself believe (which may, among a group of medical men, sound like heresy) that the most complete extension of clinical services, if the effort stopped there, would reverse the population trend of the sad, lost tribes. I do believe that with a clinical attention twice as adequate as we are able to give now, plus health education, which we can not give now, plus economic hope, the tide could be turned. (Collier 1933:62)

The "anthropological approach" as applied to health was perhaps most obvious in *The Navajo Door* by Alexander and Dorothea Leighton (1944), an introduction to the health beliefs and practices of the Navajos written especially for Indian Bureau employees providing medical care. The message in part was that Navajo ceremonials, while not adequate therapy for appendicitis or tuberculosis, did have great psychotherapeutic and social value; traditional healers were to be respected as potentially valuable allies; and great care needed to be taken with interpreters who could be of enormous help as health educators if properly trained. This attitude was in marked contrast with that of many physicians and others in the Indian Bureau who believed that medicine men were the enemies of progress and the ones standing in the way of adequate hospital and health care utilization by most Navajos. Tillim (1936:355) wrote:

The real harm caused by these men comes from the perpetuation of superstitions and failure to recognize the limits of their usefulness as healers. . . . It is my conviction that they are to blame for much crippling and many deaths which could be averted by proper medical care. Time and again they call for physicians when the patients are about to die; the reason for calling a doctor at the last moment is to have an opportunity to shift the blame, or to gain the help of the agency or the local missionary for the burial. (See also Schnur 1942)

By way of contrast, the Leightons wrote:

> When it comes to hospitalization of Navahos, one sometimes meets with a surprising amount of resistance. It is well to bear in mind that the Indians' experience with hospitals extends over a period of less than one lifetime. Only recently have they brought in a patient before he was moribund; they commonly hold the opinion that a hospital is a place to go to die. A generation ago this was the view of most people in our culture and it still is the view of many people today. (Leighton and Leighton 1944:56)

Considering the descriptions of Navajo service facilities cited previously, the Navajos' resistance may have been based upon an entirely accurate perception of the fate likely to befall them in hospital.

Employment of medical staff increased throughout the Indian Service during the Depression, largely because employment opportunities elsewhere had become limited, as well as because the Indian New Deal really was committed to improving a variety of services. The number of Navajo hospital beds increased during this period also, from 352 in 1933 to 564 in 1940. The latter year was the high water mark, however. With entry of the United States into World War II, money and personnel were diverted to the military; several hospitals were closed, and of those that remained in 1943 only the one at Fort Defiance (with 250 beds) had more than one physician. Judging by these data, there were about ten physicians serving the Navajos during the war years (Leighton and Leighton 1944:48).

To implement the postwar policy of terminating the special legal status of Indians, the Hoover Commission made several recommendations with regard to the provision of health care. These included the following:

1. Responsibility for public health functions for Indians should be transferred to state and local governments wherever possible.

2. Responsibility for medical care of destitute Indians should be transferred to state or county authorities.

3. The Indian Service should establish a schedule of medical care and hospital fees and should collect from all Indians who are able to pay.

4. The present use of contracts with qualified private physicians in or adjacent to Indian communities to provide medical service for Indian people should be further developed as a step in the transition to a normal plan of medical care.

5. Indian Service general hospitals should be turned over to county or state governments or to voluntary community hospital associations, to be operated as nonprofit hospitals for the people of the community, including the Indians.

6. The large off-reservation Indian Service hospitals, which take chiefly tuberculosis patients from a wide area and which offer specialized service that most reservation hospitals do not provide, should continue to be administered by the Bureau of Indian Affairs until satisfactory arrangements can be made for their operation by state or local governments (USPHS 1957:272).

Several task forces organized by the American Medical Association reported on health conditions among Navajos during the late 1940s (Woods 1947; Moorman 1949). The issue of divesting the Bureau of Indian Affairs of its health-related responsibilities was mentioned only in passing. In general, very strong recommendations were made regarding the improvement of services. Without doubt they could not have been acted upon by local government authorities. The Hoover Commission recommendations with regard to health care were of a piece with the recommendations regarding changes in Indian policy more generally and reflected a conservative reaction to the New Deal programs. Even an organization as politically conservative as the AMA, however, which would have been expected to support the Hoover Commission's recommendations with respect to shifting Indian health care increasingly into the private sector, said essentially nothing about the desirability of such a change. Indeed, as noted above, the task force recommendations called for such extensive improvements in the provision of services that only the federal government would have been in a position to implement them (see Foard 1950; Pijoan and McCammon 1949).

The clear intent of the Commission was to strip the Bureau of its authority and integrate Indians into the larger society. Lacking state or county willingness to assume responsibility for their health care, however, it was believed that this responsibility should be transferred to the U.S. Public Health Service. In addition to the Hoover Commission, a number of other organizations supported the transfer: the Association of State and Territorial Physicians, the Governor's Interstate Council on Indian Affairs, the American Public Health Association, the National Tuberculosis Association, and the Association on American Indian Affairs. Predictably, the Bureau of Indian Affairs opposed the change.

A number of reasons were offered for the transfer. First, the recruitment of staff would improve because the benefits for personnel were better in the PHS than in the BIA. Second, professional medical supervision would replace lay control of health programs. Third, the full resources of the Public Health Service could be brought to bear on problems of Indian health. Fourth, the Public Health Service might be more successful in obtaining appropriations for health programs. Fifth, the duplication of health-related efforts might be diminished. Sixth, the Public Health Service was thought to have more direct access to state and local health authorities and to federal agencies in the Department of Health, Education and Welfare that made grants to states for health-related purposes (USPHS 1957). The improvement of health was seen as a prerequisite to the termination of the Indians' special status. Finally, of course, transfer would weaken the hegemony of the Bureau of Indian Affairs.

Transfer of responsibility from the Bureau of Indian Affairs to the Public Health Service occurred in 1955.[1] The consequences with respect to hospital utilization by Navajos are displayed in table 5.2. A few deficiencies in the data must be noted. First, the number of hospital beds refers only to government facilities on the reservation. Not included are mission hospitals—which were not large in any event—and off-reservation contract and referral hospitals, most notably tuberculosis sanatoria to which increasing numbers of patients were sent beginning in 1952. Thus, the effective bed/ population ratio was probably higher than these figures suggest.

Second, the population estimates are probably lower than the actual service population because they do not include all the Navajos living in off-reservation communities who made use of

TABLE 5.2
Hospital Utilization, 1940–1979

Year	Est. pop.	No. beds in area hospitals	Beds per 1,000 pop.	No. admissions Navajo area hosp.	No. admissions All Res. Navajos to all hospitals	Admissions per 1,000 pop. Area	Admissions per 1,000 pop. All Res. Navajos	Avg. length of stay Area hosp.	Avg. length of stay All Res. Navajos	Occupancy rates, area hospitals Reported	Occupancy rates, area hospitals Calculated
1940	50,000	564	11.3	9,142		182.8		20.5			50
1955	80,000–82,000	432	5.3	6,620		81.7		14–16		72.5	
1960	80,000–90,000	427	4.7–5.3	10,641		118–133		13.1			89.4
1966	92,000–105,000	547	5.2–5.9	16,673		158–181				83.6	
1972				18,127	21,497				8.9		
1973	130,000	547	4.2	18,286	22,060	140	170		8.6	69	
1974				18,111	21,536				6.3		
1975				18,097	21,217				6.3		
1976				19,472	22,052			5.8	5.8		56
1977	139,000			18,449	22,921	132	164		5.6	60	
1978	142,000	557	3.9								
1979					21,539		152		5.4		

*Calculated as follows:

$$\frac{\text{No. area hospital admissions} \times \text{avg. length of stay}}{\text{No. beds} \times 365} = \frac{\text{No. patient days}}{\text{No. available beds days}} = \text{Occupancy rate}$$

the reservation facilities and may underestimate the reservation population as well.

Third, the table is difficult to read because different figures apply to the same variable. For instance, under the category of number of admissions, I have listed admissions to federal hospitals on the reservation as reported in various government documents, as well as the admissions of all Navajos giving a reservation address regardless of hospital location. The latter are based upon my analysis of USPHS computerized discharge data. Similarly, admissions per 1,000 population are based upon the two different sets of admissions figures; and average length of stay is given both for patients in reservation hospitals and for all reservation-resident Navajo patients regardless of hospital. Clearly, the figures for all hospitalized Navajos giving a reservation address are more complete than those based upon admissions to government hospitals on the reservation. From 1972 to 1977, both sets of data are available and show that the pattern of admissions is parallel; that is to say, the numbers are relatively constant from one year to the next.

Finally, the table shows occupancy rates for government hospitals on the reservation. The figures in the first column are from government and tribal publications. The second column figures are calculated using the formula at the bottom of the table. I did this to give a better picture of hospital utilization. The discrepancy of four percentage points between the rate calculated for 1976 and that reported for 1977 suggests that I have not introduced significant distortions.

Despite these problems, the table establishes the general pattern. The number of available beds declined from 1940 to 1955 and then began to increase after transfer to the Public Health Service. Manpower also increased: from 16 physicians in 1950 to 23 in 1955, 37 in 1958 (TNY 1958:334), 43 in 1960, and 115 in 1977 (Navajo Health Systems Agency 1978:232).

Utilization patterns shifted markedly in response to changes in services and diseases. The decline in average length of stay was due largely to the decline in tuberculosis. After 1952, many of the tuberculosis patients would not have contributed to these figures because they were hospitalized elsewhere, but in 1960 the average stay of the 58 tuberculosis patients hospitalized at the Fort Defiance sanatorium was 115.6 days, compared to stays of

5.6 to 13.3 days for nontuberculosis patients at Navajo area hosptials (TNY 1961:91).

Decline in average length of stay cannot be attributed solely to the disappearance of tuberculosis. Table 5.3 shows that from 1972 through 1978 it dropped in every diagnostic category. Table 5.4 indicates that the decline occurred for every age group as well.

I shall deal with average length of stay in more detail below. For the present the reader's attention is directed back to table 5.2 where data on number of hospitalizations and occupancy rates are displayed. Notice that the number of hospitalizations decreased from 1940 through 1955, almost doubled between 1955 and 1960, and then increased again during the 1960s. Throughout the 1970s the number remained essentially unchanged whether one considers only Navajo area hospitals or Navajos hospitalized regardless of location. Admissions per 1,000 population followed a similar course, declining between 1940 and 1955, increasing from 1955 through the 1960s, and declining slowly through the 1970s.

Occupancy rates have fluctuated widely over the past forty-five to fifty years. In 1933 the rate was 111 percent (see table 5.1). Seven years later after the construction of over 200 new beds, it was down to about 50 percent (see table 5.2). After the war the rate increased to about 72 percent as the number of beds fell by 130. It continued to increase from 1955 through the 1960s even as the number of beds increased. By the early 1970s, the rate had begun to decline as the number of beds and admissions leveled off and average length of stay continued to decline.

The health services literature is generally concerned with the impact of the health care system—financing, organization, and manpower—on utilization. Population characteristics receive less attention. In the following discussion, however, I shall maintain that characteristics of the health care system as well as those of the Navajo population best explain changing patterns of hospital utilization. These characteristics have to do with federal Indian policy, disease patterns, the effectiveness of therapy, and Navajo social organization and the role of the hospital.

With regard to Indian policy and the availability of services, it cannot be accidental that the number of hospital admissions dropped so dramatically between 1940 and 1955 and rebounded

TABLE 5.3

LENGTH OF HOSPITAL STAY AND PROPORTIONATE DISTRIBUTION BY DIAGNOSTIC CATEGORY
(All Navajo Hospitalizations)

Diagnosis	1972		1973		1974		1975		1976		1977		1978	
	LOS	% dischrgs.	LOS	% dischrgs.	LOS	% dischrgs.	LOS	% dischrgs.	LOS	% dischrgs.	LOS	% dischrgs.	LOS	% dischrgs.
I infective & parasitic	12.5	4.31	7.9	3.90	6.9	3.43	7.3	3.38	5.4	5.00	5.8	3.46	5.2	2.76
II neoplasms	11.6	1.08	8.4	.89	8.4	1.09	9.3	1.12	8.4	1.03	7.5	1.21	7.9	1.18
III endocr. nutr. metab.	13.5	.94	10.5	.96	10.5	.98	10.4	.90	8.1	1.20	7.9	1.12	7.1	1.16
IV blood & blood forming	10.8	.55	8.9	.59	8.4	.54	6.5	.40	5.5	.49	6.4	.47	7.3	.36
V mental	15.8	2.94	26.9	2.58	13.6	2.28	17.0	2.38	9.7	2.43	7.0	2.26	6.2	2.60
VI nervous system	10.2	4.94	9.4	4.58	6.8	4.65	6.9	4.78	6.3	4.17	7.7	3.84	5.6	4.50
VII circulatory	12.5	1.88	14.2	1.84	9.2	2.12	8.7	1.89	8.8	2.02	9.0	1.92	9.1	1.95
VIII respiratory	8.8	9.53	9.0	9.12	6.9	8.67	6.6	8.32	6.1	6.68	5.5	7.19	5.8	7.19
IX digestive	12.3	4.58	9.5	4.76	8.3	4.93	8.5	5.19	8.6	5.14	8.5	5.13	8.4	5.32
X genitourinary	11.5	4.43	12.5	4.31	7.9	3.78	8.5	3.78	7.9	3.83	8.1	3.89	7.5	4.19
XI pregnancy & childbirth	5.0	18.81	4.6	19.80	3.6	20.43	3.4	20.86	3.4	19.58	3.3	21.06	3.3	21.05

XII skin & subcutan.	13.9	2.03	9.9	2.20	7.8	2.44	9.0	2.28	9.9	3.06	7.7	2.62	8.2	2.33
XIII musculo-skeletal	14.6	1.53	17.0	1.63	10.4	1.56	11.1	1.53	9.8	1.65	10.0	1.52	9.6	1.58
XIV congenital	12.4	1.00	9.7	2.09	8.0	1.92	7.4	1.79	6.0	1.81	7.0	2.07	7.4	2.04
XV perinatal morb. mort.	9.1	2.89	8.3	3.05	7.0	3.37	6.8	2.96	7.2	2.33	5.7	2.75	4.5	3.71
XVI ill-defined	9.5	6.71	8.7	6.80	6.9	6.89	7.1	7.62	6.9	7.42	5.9	7.81	6.8	7.41
XVII accidents	9.7	15.53	10.7	16.21	8.4	14.59	7.9	13.74	7.1	13.76	7.2	13.90	6.5	14.31
XVIII missing DX	5.0	15.23	4.4	14.68	3.1	16.32	3.1	17.10	3.1	18.39	3.4	17.77	3.2	16.36
ℓLOS	8.9		8.6		6.3		6.3		5.8		5.6		5.4	
Total discharges	25,292		25,987		25,852		25,239		26,107		27,027		25,726	

TABLE 5.4
AVERAGE LENGTH OF HOSPITAL STAY OF NAVAJOS RESIDENT ON THE
RESERVATION, BY AGE, 1972–1979 (NEWBORNS NOT INCLUDED)

Age	1972	1973	1974	1975	1976	1977	1978	1979
< 1	11.1	9.2	8.3	7.5	7.2	6.6	7.2	6.2
1–4	11.7	9.0	6.0	5.6	5.3	5.2	5.5	4.8
5–9	6.7	7.8	4.8	5.9	4.7	5.1	4.2	4.7
10–19	7.7	7.0	5.8	5.6	4.9	4.5	4.8	4.3
20–29	7.4	7.5	5.3	5.4	4.7	4.5	4.4	4.2
30–39	10.5	9.7	7.0	7.4	6.1	6.0	5.5	5.0
40–49	11.1	11.6	8.1	7.6	8.0	7.5	6.8	7.1
50–59	13.2	12.2	8.9	10.3	9.1	8.9	8.5	8.4
60–64	17.0	14.5	10.0	8.8	8.4	8.2	9.5	8.5
65–69	11.8	15.6	9.6	9.5	8.5	10.9	10.0	9.6
70–74	14.6	15.5	10.1	11.1	10.8	9.4	10.6	9.8
>75	18.0	16.8	11.5	11.7	12.8	11.7	9.6	9.9

so rapidly after transfer to the Public Health Service in 1955. Though there is some evidence that crude mortality rates and infant, maternal, and tuberculosis deaths all declined from 1940 to the mid-1950s, it does not seem likely that this was the cause of the decline in utilization. If it were, the rate of utilization should not have risen so quickly in the late 1950s and 1960s. Conversely, the fact that admissions reached a plateau in the 1970s cannot be well explained by changes in the availability of services. It is true that the number of beds remained essentially constant and the number of beds per 1,000 population therefore declined slightly, but occupancy rates declined during this period. This would seem to indicate that it was not limited availability of beds that caused the decline.

In the early 1970s a shortage of nurses resulted in closing some beds in the Shiprock hospital (McKenzie 1974). The number of nurses per bed, however, increased dramatically from 1955 to the present (see Table 5.5). Acute local shortages do not explain the reservation pattern.

The data in chapter 3 leave no doubt that disease patterns have changed significantly over the past forty years. As table 5.6 indicates, the change is reflected in shifting patterns of discharge diagnoses from both federal and contract hospitals in 1959,

TABLE 5.5

NURSING STAFF, NAVAJO RESERVATION, 1950–1978

Year	RNs		PHN		LPNs		Nursing asst.		RN/Bed
	Total Positions	Unfilled	Total	Unfilled	Total	Unfilled	Total	Unfilled	
1950[a]	62	unknown	8	unknown	unknown	unknown	unknown	unknown	unknown
1955[a,b]	64	unknown	24	unknown	unknown	unknown	70	unknown	.14
1960[b]	94	unknown	28	unknown	unknown	unknown	88	unknown	.22
1977[c]	266	31	39	0	160	10	78	2	.42[d]
1978[c]	281	21	47	1	142	3	141	2	.46[d]

[a]TNY 1958
[b]TNY 1961
[c]Navajo Health Authority Manpower Surveys 1977, 1978
[d]Filled positions only

TABLE 5.6
DISTRIBUTION OF DIAGNOSES OF MAJOR CAUSES OF HOSPITALIZATION,
NAVAJO AREA HOSPITALS, 1959–1977
(NEWBORNS AND DELIVERIES OMITTED)

Diagnosis	1959		1968		1977	
	#	%	#	%	#	%
Influenza and pneumonia	1,049	10.8	1,746	11.6	942	5.8
Tuberculosis	195	2.0	225	1.5	130	0.8
Dysentary and gastroenteritis	776	8.0	998	6.7	218	1.3
Subtotal	2,050	21.2	2,969	19.9	1,290	8.0
Circulatory	229	2.3	387	2.6	512	3.2
Accidents	1,488	15.4	2,751	18.4	2,947	18.3
Neoplasms	147	1.5	238	1.6	440	2.7
Total, all discharges	9,679		14,945		16,098	

1968, and 1977. Though the number of hospitalizations increased from one year to the next, infectious diseases decreased relatively and in the second period absolutely. In each instance the numbers increased from 1959 through 1968, probably as hospital utilization increased, and then declined dramatically starting in the late 1960s even as hospitalizations for all causes remained essentially unchanged. Although the number of admissions resulting from accidents almost doubled, however, they did not greatly increase their relative contribution to hospitalizations. Accidents increased most rapidly in the 1960s and tended to reach a plateau in the 1970s. The incidence and severity of infectious diseases have been decreasing, and man-made, psychosocial, and degenerative diseases have replaced them only partially as a cause of hospitalization.

The decline in respiratory and gastrointestinal diseases has had its most obvious impact on children. According to discharge data from Navajo area IHS hospitals from 1959 through 1977 (table 5.7), between 1959 and 1968 the number of admissions in all age groups increased substantially, and the proportionate age distribution of patients remained essentially unchanged. Beginning in the late 1960s, the rate of increase of admissions began to decline and the number of pediatric admissions actually de-

TABLE 5.7
DISCHARGES, NAVAJO AREA INDIAN HEALTH SERVICE HOSPITALS,
SELECTED YEARS AND AGE GROUPS
(EXCLUDING NEWBORNS)

Age	1959 #	1959 %	1968 #	1968 %	1974 #	1974 %	1977 #	1977 %
≤10	3,156	32.5	4,854	29.1	4,572	25.5	4,087	22.0
≥65	595	6.1	1,195	7.2	1,350	7.4	1,501	8.1
Total discharges	9,708		16,688		17,906		18,616	

creased. However, the number of admissions of people aged 65 and older continued to increase, though at a slow rate. The result has been a shift in the age distribution of patients, such that by 1977 patients under 10 years of age (excluding newborns) were only 22 percent of the total, compared to 32 percent in 1959.

The degree to which medical therapy has influenced mortality, morbidity, and utilization was discussed in chapter 3. I believe therapy had a substantial impact upon tuberculosis and maternal mortality (diseases affecting mainly adults) and therefore had an impact on utilization. It is less clear what the impact upon infant and child mortality has been, but it is likely that environmental improvements were distinctly more important than medical care. No matter what the cause, a decline is reflected in diminished utilization by the pediatric age group.

The leveling off of hospital admissions in the 1970s may have resulted from the increased utilization of outpatient services for the earlier treatment of illnesses that otherwise would have led to hospitalization. Outpatient treatment may also have led to increased willingness to shorten hospital stays since it created greater assurance of follow-up care in hospital and field clinics. Both may be considered aspects of the impact of medical therapy. As table 5.8 indicates, outpatient utilization has increased substantially over the past forty years and did not reach a plateau in the 1970s as did inpatient utilization.

The relationship between clinic and hospital utilization may be examined more closely using the synchronic data in table 5.9. If the hypothesis that outpatient visits cause hospitalizations to decline is correct, then one would expect to see an inverse relationship between average clinic visits per person and hos-

TABLE 5.8
OUTPATIENT VISITS, NAVAJO RESERVATION, 1940–1978

Year	No. Visits	Visits/person (approximate)	Source
1940	54,403	1.1	Navajo Medical News 1940
1955–1956 (2 yr. average)	36,448.2	0.5	USPHS 1957:255
1960	138,210	1.5–1.7	TNY 1961:93
1971	436,072		Navajo Health Systems Agency, 1978, I:411; and Navajo Area I.H.S. 1979*b*
1972	454,291		
1973	469,047	3.6	
1974	missing data		
1975	537,573		
1976	581,640		
1977	588,180		
1978	635,808	4.5	

pitalization rates per 1,000 population (using Indian Health Service catchment areas as the populations). In fact, no relationship whatever exists between the two variables (Spearman's rho = 0.38). Visits per person are inversely related to the population per clinic (Spearman's rho = −0.5); that is to say, the greater the number of people for each clinic, the lower the average number of clinic visits per person. The average distance from a hospital is inversely related to the hospitalization rate (Spearman's rho = −0.55). These crude data indicate that clinic visits and hospitalizations vary independently and are related to the availability of facilities.

Moreover, when the relationship between average length of stay and clinic visits per person is examined, no significant relationship is observed (Spearman's rho = 0.28 corrected for ties). Thus, at this level of analysis I cannot demonstrate that the increasing utilization of clinics is related to either lower rates of hospital utilization or shortened lengths of stay. It must be conceded, however, that this is but a crude test of the hypothesis, and much more refined data would be necessary to test it adequately.

TABLE 5.9
Hospital and Clinic Utilization, Navajo Reservation, F.Y. 1976

Service unit	Population	No. clinic visits	Visits per person	Population per clinic	No. hospital discharges	Hospital rate per 1,000	Miles to nearest hospital	Avg. length of stay
Chinle	22,972	110,880	4.8	1,276	3,087	134	64	6.3
Crownpoint	11,553	67,707	5.9	888	2,264	196	33	6.5
Ft. Defiance	17,195	90,363	5.3	2,456	2,881	168	36	6.1
Gallup	18,538	90,505	4.9	1,685	3,822	206	28	6.1
Kayenta	12,493	53,552	4.3	2,082	1,176	94	59	6.3
Shiprock	29,152	98,378	3.4	2,242	4,413	151	46	5.2
Tuba City	12,628	72,440	5.7	1,578	2,485	197	38	5.1
Winslow	9,941	45,756	4.6	1,656	2,641	266	56	4.7

Source: Navajo Health Systems Agency 1978, 1:250

*Estimated from Davis and Kunitz (1978)

Improved therapy has increased the acceptability of hospitalization. Hospitals are no longer regarded as places in which to die, since patients generally survive their stays there. The Navajos are pragmatic and willing to adopt innovations that promise some benefit, and hospital care is such an innovation. As early as 1905 one observer remarked: "Their faith in our system of medical treatment has increased. They readily yield to surgical treatment" (Commissioner of Indian Affairs 1905:142). And on her inspection trip through the reservation in the mid-1920s, Gregg (1965) reported being asked by two elderly Navajos if they could have a surgeon assigned to their hospital rather than an internist. By that time sterile technique and anesthesia had made surgery much more effective than most modes of nonsurgical treatment, with the exception perhaps of vaccination, immunization, and diphtheria antitoxin.

The increased use of hospitals for childbirth may also reflect a growing perception of their safety. Indeed, not only did maternal mortality decline because hospital utilization increased, but hospital utilization increased because maternal mortality declined—that is to say, because hospitals became safer places in which to have babies.

Related to much of the foregoing as well as to changes in Navajo social organization is the fact that the social function of the hospital has been changing. Once again I shall use multiple regression analysis and consider several different dependent variables which reflect different aspects of utilization: average hospitalization rate, age of patients, and use of procedures of equal complexity but different levels of urgency. The point I shall make is that in each case population characteristics such as proportion of income derived from wage work are important determinants of hospital utilization. Consider first average annual hospitalization rates in 1972–1976 (see table 5.10). Using a model with only one independent variable, the best predictor is distance from the nearest hospital (R^2 = 24 percent). The best two-variable model includes both distance and the proportion of men working 50 to 52 weeks (R^2 = 46 percent). The best three-variable model adds household size (R^2 = 66 percent).

Of special note is the fact that average educational level of male heads of households is highly correlated (r = 0.73) with the proportion working 50 to 52 weeks. The high correlation be-

TABLE 5.10

COEFFICIENTS OF DETERMINATION, R^2, FOR THE FIRST AND EACH
CONSECUTIVE PREDICTOR (VARIABLE PRESENTED IN ORDER OF ENTRANCE)

Dependent Variable:

Average number of hospitalizations (1972–1976) per 1,000 people

Variable	R^2	Regression coefficients	Standard error
NEARH	.2363	−1.307**	0.325
HSIZE	.4647	−1.694*	0.599
WORKM	.6599	−0.201**	0.050

For the 3-variable model, F = 9.03 and PROB F = 0.0014

*$p < 0.05$

**$p < 0.001$

tween these two independent variables means that it is difficult to distinguish between their effects. Neither distance and employment ($r = -0.24$) nor distance and education ($r = -0.42$) is strongly correlated, suggesting that the effects of distance and employment/education are indeed distinguishable.

In the two-variable model when distance is controlled, full-time employment is inversely related to hospitalization: the higher the proportion of men working full-time, the lower the hospital discharge rate. Because employment is so highly correlated with education as well as with per capita income and the availability of such domestic conveniences as electricity, running water, and bathrooms, it is probable that the health of the families of wage workers is better than the health of other people. The result is lower hospitalization rates.

Household size contributes about 20 percent to the variance in hospitalization rates. That is, controlling for distance and employment, the larger the average household size in a district, the lower the hospitalization rate. I suggest that where households are smaller there will be fewer kin available to care for a sick family member, and hospitals will be increasingly relied upon. In this model, household size makes a contribution independent of reliance on full-time wage work. To the degree, however, that wage work results in the weakening of kin ties, changes may occur in the way formal institutions such as hospitals are used. As these data are at the aggregate level, I can do no more than suggest the possibility. Field studies are necessary to confirm what for now must remain a reasonable hypothesis.

I have shown that the elderly represent a slowly increasing proportion of the hospitalized population. The situation of the elderly has been of increasing concern to a variety of tribal and health and welfare workers on the reservation (Lyon 1978; York 1979). In response to decreased hospital utilization by the pediatric age group and emigration of young adults from rural areas, hospitals are becoming places that increasingly provide care many believe might be more appropriately provided either in the home or in extended care facilities. In a multiple regression analysis with mean age of patients from each land management district as the dependent variable (see table 5.11), the best single-variable model includes distance from the nearest hospital providing surgery as the independent variable ($R^2 = 22$ percent): the greater the distance, the older the patients.

TABLE 5.11
COEFFICIENTS OF DETERMINATION, R^2, FOR EACH CONSECUTIVE MODEL
(VARIABLES PRESENTED IN ORDER OF ENTRANCE)

Regression: Mean Age of Patients

Variable	R^2	Regression coefficients	Standard error
NEARS	.2164	0.027*	0.011
WELF	.3778	−0.013*	0.005
AMHH	.5222	1.137*	0.296
WAGE → WELF	.6214	0.024**	0.005
EDM → NEARS	.6232	−0.134*	0.054

(→) replaces: Final model F = 7.72   PROB F = 0.0028
*$p < 0.05$
**$p < 0.001$

The best two-variable model adds proportion of income from welfare and explains 38 percent of the variance. Controlling for distance, the lower the proportion of income derived from welfare, the older the patients.

Two three-variable models are about equally effective, each explaining 62 percent of the variance. The first includes distance from surgery, substitutes wage work for welfare (the higher the proportion of income from wage work, the older the patients), and adds average age of male household heads. Controlling for distance and dependence on wage work, the older the male household heads, the greater the average age of patients. The second model is the same as the first but substitutes average educational level of male household heads for distance from surgery. The greater the educational level, the lower the age of patients.

On the face of it, it is not surprising that distance from surgery should be related to age of patients. The hospitals that provide surgery tend to be in communities in which wage work is relatively available and which attract young adults from the rural hinterlands, leaving behind a residual older population. However, distance and age of male and female heads of households are not correlated. Unfortunately, inadequate population data do not permit the calculation of age-specific hospitalization rates. There is some evidence from the third variable, average age of male household heads, that when distance and source of income are controlled, the age of the population is significantly related to the average age of patients. Distance from surgery may not be a substitution variable for age, therefore, but may instead be related to isolation, perhaps to the fact that when older people from more remote areas fall ill they are brought to hospitals because home health services cannot reach them rapidly.

The fact that dependence on welfare is related to lower average age of patients and dependence on wage work to higher average age supports the hypothesis suggested above in respect of kin networks and involvement in wage work. Where dependence upon wage work is relatively great, family organization may be such that older people who fall ill will have no one to care for them at home. Conversely, dependence upon welfare is related to low participation in the wage economy and may be related to the maintenance of strong cooperative patterns among kin, which may make possible the maintenance of older people at home (once the factor of isolation is taken into account).

If hospitals are increasingly being used to care for elderly people who cannot be maintained at home, it would be expected that the average length of stay of people aged 65 and older might be increasing. Table 5.4 shows this not to be the case. When this age category is examined more carefully by land management district, however, a more complex picture emerges (see table 5.12). Between 1972 and 1978, the only land management districts in which average length of stay of older people increased were 1, 2, and 3, all on the western end of the reservation in the area served by the Tuba City hospital. Elsewhere it declined, sometimes very substantially.

TABLE 5.12
AVERAGE LENGTH OF STAY BY LAND MANAGEMENT DISTRICT FOR
PEOPLE 65 YEARS AND OLDER

LMD	1972	1973	1974	1975	1976	1977	1978
1	8.4	9.5	9.3	9.4	11.5	9.6	8.9
2	5.5	7.1	12.2	7.1	13.1	16.3	9.3
3	9.3	9.0	8.1	14.2	8.0	11.7	12.1
4	12.3	14.8	10.7	8.7	12.1	13.6	8.0
5	10.1	8.3	6.8	5.9	11.4	17.5	10.0
7	9.0	7.6	7.6	8.8	8.1	9.1	8.6
8	12.7	12.0	9.3	8.7	12.1	11.5	11.3
9	21.4	16.6	9.2	11.5	17.0	9.6	10.2
10	15.1	28.9	15.3	12.5	12.4	10.8	10.3
11	17.6	24.3	12.9	16.4	15.6	9.7	14.1
12	17.7	14.7	12.2	10.9	11.8	9.4	8.9
13	49.9	14.0	13.5	12.9	10.6	6.4	10.4
14	11.3	13.7	12.4	8.8	8.2	8.7	10.7
15	14.6	12.0	11.2	12.1	10.4	11.3	9.9
16	17.7	14.3	12.0	12.0	10.1	10.7	11.7
17	21.2	18.5	10.5	11.4	11.8	10.1	9.3
18	15.7	20.7	12.3	12.0	13.3	13.7	8.6
19	14.4	18.3	10.8	8.3	9.1	7.3	8.4
On Res. (total)	15.1	14.6	10.8	11.0	11.1	10.6	9.9
Off Res.	13.1	19.5	9.2	13.1	11.3	13.4	10.1

In chapter 2 it was shown that there have been consistent differences from the eastern to the western ends of the reservation with regard to economic and demographic patterns. The population in the west has had higher rates of emigration than the population in the east, and it is possible that those districts in which the elderly have increasing lengths of stay are the ones in which there are fewer young people available to care for the elderly. Furthermore, judging by the very long hospitalizations reported from some of the eastern districts in the early 1970s and then followed by a rapid decline through 1978, nursing homes may have become increasingly available there, relieving hospitals of the necessity of long-term admissions.

Changes in the health care system have also influenced changes in hospital utilization patterns of elderly people. In 1975, a new 125-bed hospital was opened in Tuba City, replacing a 75-bed hospital. The design of the new hospital was based upon utilization patterns from the 1960s, at which time pediatric admissions were higher than they became in the 1970s. Thus the pediatric wards were not utilized as heavily as had been expected, and beds were available for use by other age groups. The result seems to have been that average length of stay for the elderly increased in districts 1, 2, and 3 and decreased elsewhere during the 1970s. By 1978 average length of stay was essentially the same across the reservation. This suggests that hospital characteristics rather than patient demand were of most significance in explaining the observed patterns of length of stay.

Both population and hospital characteristics are therefore important in explaining utilization, the relative importance of each being dependent upon that aspect of utilization being examined. As demonstrated in chapters 2 and 3, tubal ligations, induced abortions, and Caesarean sections are better explained by population characteristics than by hospital accessibility. Overall hospitalization rates, however, are better explained by accessibility. Hospital utilization by the elderly is more ambiguous.

To explore these relationships more closely I have examined three surgical procedures: cholecystectomies, appendectomies, and hysterectomies. Table 5.13 indicates the relative ranking of these procedures (along with eight others) in terms of complexity, urgency, and necessity. Notice that the three chosen (for which there were adequate numbers for analysis) did not vary much in complexity (ranks 6, 5, and 4 for appendectomies, cholecystectomies, and hysterectomies, respectively), whereas appendectomies were the most urgent and necessary, followed by cholecystectomies and hysterectomies.

The reasoning behind this analysis is the following. I have shown that the predictors of hospitalization vary depending upon the outcome measure being considered. Hospitalizations

TABLE 5.13
INDEXES OF COMPLEXITY, URGENCY AND NECESSITY
OF 11 SELECTED PROCEDURES

	Complexity	Urgency	Necessity
Appendectomy	6	1	1
Cataract	3	11	2.5
Hernia repair	8	5	2.5
Prostatectomy	2	4	4
Cholecystectomy	5	3	5
Dilation & curettage (exc. abortion)	10	2	6
Hemorrhoidectomy	9	7	7
Varicose vein stripping	7	10	8
Lumbar laminectomy (for disk)	1	6	9
Hysterectomy	4	8	10
Tonsillectomy	11	9	11

Source: Bombardier et al. 1977

may be discretionary or nondiscretionary, and I hypothesize that population characteristics—especially measures of modernization—will be especially important as predictors of discretionary procedures. Recall that in chapter 3 it was suggested that such procedures are especially likely to be used by those who are most acculturated. The examination of these three operations is another attempt to examine that possibility, as well as to consider the larger point that the use of hospitals is changing as disease patterns shift, such that urgent admissions become less common. Once more the reader is reminded that aggregate data are being used to make inferences about individual behavior.

Cholecystectomy. Gallbladder disease has been observed to be unusually common among American Indians, including Navajos (Nelson et al. 1971; Lam 1954; Sievers and Marquis 1962; Comess et al. 1967; Thistle et al. 1971; Sampliner et al. 1970). The data from 1972 to 1978 (see table 5.14) are similar to those reported by Nelson et al. (1971) from the Fort Defiance Hospital in 1966 to 1968 in the following respects: women outnumber men (4.6:1 in their study, 3.1:1 in mine), and women are operated on at an earlier age than men.

In discussing the ratio of women to men, Nelson et al. (1971)

TABLE 5.14
AGE, SEX, AND NUMBER OF CHOLECYSTECTOMY
PATIENTS, NAVAJO RESERVATION

Year	Men Mean age	Men Median age	Number	Women Mean age	Women Median age	Number
1972	56.4	56.0	50	43.5	39.0	145
1973	53.1	52.5	59	39.7	37.0	149
1974	51.3	50.0	46	39.6	37.0	163
1975	50.2	49.0	58	40.1	38.0	192
1976	50.4	47.0	62	41.1	39.0	205
1977	54.6	54.0	59	42.1	36.0	206
1978	53.7	49.0	69	40.2	36.5	201

indicated that 4.6:1 is higher than is found in many other populations. Ratios among other Southwestern tribes were found to vary between 3:1 and 7:1, whereas ratios among non-Indians varied from 2:1 to 3:1. The fact that the ratio observed here is so much lower than the one they reported may have to do with the number of years and size of the population for which data were available or with changing utilization patterns. Changes in the disease itself are not likely in so short a period.

Because gallbladder disease is so common among Navajos, I thought that access to care and measures of involvement in the modern wage economy might prove to be unrelated to the incidence of gallbladder surgery. On the contrary, table 5.15 indicates that the best single predictor is distance from surgery: the

TABLE 5.15
COEFFICIENTS OF DETERMINATIONS, R^2, FOR EACH CONSECUTIVE MODEL:
VARIOUS SURGICAL PROCEDURES

Dependent variable	Independent variables	R^2	Regression coefficients	Standard error
Cholecystectomy	NEARS	.4938	−0.007*	0.003
	BATH	.6131	0.002*	0.001
Appendectomy	BATH	.2585	0.005*	0.002
	HOGAN	.4624	0.005*	0.001

*$p < 0.05$
n.s. $p > 0.05$

greater the distance, the lower the rate. This explains 49 percent of the variance in the dependent variable. One of the best two-variable models adds proportion of households with bathrooms and explains 61 percent of the variance. The other equally good two-variable model substitutes average age of male household head for distance from surgery.

Appendectomy. Unlike gallbladder surgery, appendectomies occur about equally in men and women, and men are generally younger than women when they have the operation (see table 5.16). While gallbladder disease may present itself as chronic abdominal distress, appendicitis is generally thought to be a relatively acute abdominal condition requiring prompt surgical intervention. Perhaps for this reason it is not surprising that access to surgery and access to hospital are not good predictors of appendectomy rates. Table 5.15 indicates the proportion of families with an indoor bathroom is the best single predictor: the higher the proportion, the higher the rate. The best two-variable models adds proportion of families living in hogans and explains 46 percent of the variance. These two independent variables are inversely correlated (r = −.47). It is difficult to explain this pattern. It appears that measures of economic development and lack of economic development are both important, suggesting that appendicitis may be ubiquitous and neither is more important than the other as an explanatory variable. What is clear,

TABLE 5.16

AGE, SEX, AND NUMBER OF PATIENTS HAVING APPENDECTOMIES, NAVAJO RESERVATION

Year	Men Mean age	Men Median age	Number	Women Mean age	Women Median age	Number
1972	18.9	13.0	85	26.4	21.5	79
1973	20.9	15.0	128	24.1	22.0	89
1974	19.3	13.0	111	27.0	24.0	115
1975	20.9	15.0	111	25.9	25.0	119
1976	20.3	17.5	99	23.8	21.0	118
1977	21.4	16.0	87	26.5	24.0	109
1978	20.1	15.0	108	22.9	20.5	119

however, is that access to surgical care (or to any hospital) is not related to the incidence of the procedure.

Hysterectomy. The hysterectomy procedures examined excluded those usually done to remove cancerous lesions and included only ICDA codes 69.1, 69.2, and 69.4. The average age of women having this procedure is displayed in table 5.17. As a means of gaining some control over the impact of age structure, I have calculated age-specific rates per 1,000 deliveries (see table 5.18). It is clear that the rate has fluctuated from year to year with no readily discernible pattern.

TABLE 5.17
MEAN AND MEDIAN AGE OF HYSTERECTOMY PATIENTS

Fiscal year	Mean	Median	Number
1972	39.4	38.5	128
1973	38.9	38.5	71
1974	42.6	40.0	89
1975	39.7	40.0	105
1976	41.9	40.0	120
1977	42.1	40.0	79
1978	42.4	40.0	60

TABLE 5.18
AGE-SPECIFIC RATIO OF HYSTERECTOMIES/1,000 DELIVERIES

Fiscal year	15–19	20–34	35–49	Total
1972	2.2	15.1	216.2	37.4
1973	4.0	10.2	107.1	19.9
1974	0.0	7.6	159.9	22.0
1975	1.4	14.6	194.7	29.6
1976	1.4	11.7	262.8	34.4
1977	0.0	26.7	140.9	19.7
1978	0.0	5.4	158.8	17.4

The results of three regression analyses are presented in table 5.19. The first is for the crude ratio of hysterectomies per 1,000 deliveries. The best single predictor is per capita income: the higher the income, the higher the rate of hysterectomies.

TABLE 5.19

RATIO OF VAGINAL AND ABDOMINAL HYSTERECTOMIES/1,000 DELIVERIES

Dependent variable	Independent variables	R^2	Regression coefficients	Standard error
Crude Ratio	PERCAP	.3569	0.025[n.s.]	0.008
(RAVHYS)	AMHH	.4702	−1.462[n.s.]	0.816
Age 20−34	WORKM	.5250	0.027*	0.007
(ASHYS1)	WELF	.6837	0.031*	0.011
Age 35−49	WELF	.2161	−0.752*	0.232
(ASHYS2)	HOGAN	.3061	0.518*	0.232
	NEARH	.4423	1.397[n.s.]	0.756

*$p < 0.05$. All models significant at $p < .05$.

[n.s.]$p > 0.05$

The second variable is age of male household head: the greater the average age, the lower the rate.

When the ratio of hysterectomies among women ages 20 to 34 is examined, the best model includes two variables, proportion of income derived from welfare (the higher the proportion, the lower the rate), and proportion of males working full-time (the higher the proportion, the higher the rate). The two variables together explain 68 percent of the variance in the dependent variable. Thus, among younger women the variables measuring involvement in wage work best explain the ratio of hysterectomies.

Among women 35 to 49, the situation is somewhat different. Although the best one-variable model includes proportion of income from welfare (the higher the proportion, the lower the rate), it explains only 22 percent of the variance. In the two-variable model, which explains 31 percent of the variance, proportion of families living in a hogan is added: the higher the proportion, the higher the rate. The best three-variable model explains 44 percent of the variance and adds distance from the nearest hospital: the greater the distance, the greater the rate. There is a positive relationship between distance from the nearest hospital and proportion of income derived from welfare at the first order of correlation. Thus, there is some evidence that among older women in areas that are likely to have had the highest rate of fertility in the past, the rates of hysterectomies are higher than elsewhere on the reservation.

Hysterectomies have generally been performed to repair the damage of multiple deliveries, particularly uterine prolapse (Kunitz and Slocumb 1976). I was interested in the degree to which this diagnostic category was invoked as a primary indication for hysterectomy during the 1972–1978 time period. Only primary diagnoses were considered. While no trend is easily visible with respect to most major diagnostic categories, there has been a decline in the primary diagnosis of uterine prolapse which is most obvious for women 35 years of age and older. In this age group in 1972, this diagnosis was an indication for hysterectomy in 41.8 percent of the cases but in only 27.7 percent of the hysterectomy cases in 1978. For all women undergoing this procedure, the proportions with prolapse as the primary diagnoses were 33.6 and 21.5 in 1972 and 1978, respectively.

The foregoing analyses indicate that among younger Navajo women the variance in the ratio of hysterectomies is best explained by the modernization variables. Younger women may be generally more receptive to the idea of sterilization, and hysterectomy may be a method of choice to correct even minor discomforts associated with either previous births or menstruation. Among older women the degree of modernization is still important, but such factors as prevalence of gynecological problems emerge as important as well. Even in the older age category, however, the degree to which major gynecological problems are invoked as an indication for hysterectomy has been on the decline in recent years. These results are similar to those for tubal ligations, induced abortions, and Caesarean sections reported in previous chapters.

More generally these data suggest that, holding complexity of the procedure roughly constant, rates are best explained by either population or access variables, depending upon the urgency and necessity of the procedure. For hysterectomies (as well as the other gynecological procedures examined) where both urgency and necessity are relatively low, population characteristics are much more significant than hospital accessibility. For cholecystectomies where urgency and necessity are about intermediate, accessibility is far more important than population characteristics, though the latter are also significant. And for appendectomies where both urgency and necessity are high, access is unimportant and population characteristics are ambiguous. Thus, as urgency and necessity both diminish, population characteristics related to education and involvement in wage work assume greater explanatory value.

REGIONAL VARIATION IN HOSPITAL UTILIZATION

Figure 5.1 is a biplot display of several measures of hospital utilization and mortality. Not surprisingly it is similar in configuration to the analysis of variables related to mortality in figure 3.1. Districts 3, 5, and 7 in the southwestern portion of the reservation all have high rates of postneonatal mortality and hospitalization[2] and below average rates of participation in full-time wage work. Districts 10 through 18 in the east are similar in having above average mortality, relatively easy access to hospitals, and intermediate rates of hospital utilization. District 1 is fairly similar to the eastern districts, presumably as a result of the increase in wage work from the Navajo Generating Station in Page, Arizona. The upper left quadrant of the figure contains districts where hospitals are remote, utilization rates and crude mortality rates are low, and dependence upon welfare above average. The most extreme districts, 2 and 4, are contiguous in the northwestern and north-central part of the reservation. Districts 9 and 19 are farther east.

Turning attention to the variables, notice that average length of stay is positively correlated with proportion of men employed full-time. This is largely accounted for by longer-than-average hospitalizations among elderly people in districts in the east. It has been remarked above that this pattern changed in the late 1970s as average length of stay became more similar throughout the reservation.

While postneonatal and crude mortality rates are not correlated, each is correlated with average annual hospitalization rate. This suggests either that hospitals kill people or, more likely, that hospital utilization tends to be highest where the need for medical care is greatest. Almost certainly this is not related to remarkable foresight on the part of planners but to the fact that hospitals were located in areas that were centers of wage work. As noted previously, it is possible that the move to wage work has in recent years been associated with higher rates of mortality. It is also

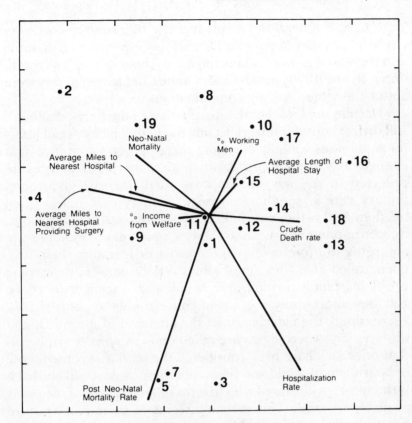

FIGURE 5.1

BIPLOT DISPLAY OF HOSPITAL UTILIZATION, MORTALITY, AND ECONOMIC
VARIABLES BY LAND MANAGEMENT DISTRICT, 1970s

possible that sick people move to be near hospitals where they can get care, but this is not likely to be of major significance in explaining the observed patterns.

DISCUSSION

Since the 1930s hospital utilization by the general United States population has increased almost threefold, and average length of hospital stay has declined (see appendix II, table 3). The pattern shows much less discontinuity than does that of the

Navajos and reflects the steady increase of insurance coverage; declining severity of episodic illnesses; improvements in therapy; and increased rates of admission for decreasingly serious conditions. By the 1970s hospitalization rates and length of stay were about the same for the two populations.

Despite the fact that the distribution of discharge diagnoses still differs considerably, reflecting the higher incidence of infectious diseases among Navajos, there is good evidence that changes in Navajo social organization and morbidity patterns are reflected in the way hospitals are used. Increasingly, discretionary care is sought as nondiscretionary care is less often needed. And as the acute infectious diseases such as tuberculosis, influenza-pneumonia, and diarrhea wane, new conditions are emerging to prominence. In the pediatric literature these have been called the "new morbidities"—behavioral and learning problems, family turmoil, and chronic and congenital disorders. But new morbidities are not of concern only to pediatricians. Increasingly the elderly attract the attention of internists; and obstetrician-gynecologists are called upon to alleviate symptoms that once may have been considered the inevitable consequence of bearing many children. In most of these cases, it is likely that it is the most acculturated who first make greatest use of the newly available services. This certainly seems to be so in respect of gynecological surgery and hospitalization of the elderly. Almost certainly these practices will diffuse more widely among Navajos in the years ahead.

But a caveat is in order. The use of services has been responsive to policy changes in the past. There is every reason to believe the same will be true in the future. Health care was increasingly available from the 1950s through the 1970s. It is becoming less readily available in the 1980s as budget cuts affect many social programs, including those of the Indian Health Service. The result may be a decline in health care utilization generally and discretionary services particularly. What the consequences for morbidity and mortality will be if this occurs, it is still too early to say.

Changing Mortality and the Role of Medicine

I BEGAN with a comparison of current mortality patterns among several different tribes and showed that as epidemic infectious diseases have waned, man-made and degenerative diseases with an important psychosocial component to their etiology have become increasingly significant. Among the tribes considered in chapter 1, there is a relationship between prereservation patterns of ecological adaptation and contemporary mortality patterns, which I explained by the degree of fit between preexisting mechanisms of social control and the demands of reservation life.

When I turned to an examination of Navajo economic and demographic patterns in chapter 2, it was to show that the stagnant reservation economy coupled with an increasingly sophisticated social service and health care system had placed a floor under the Navajos below which immiseration was unlikely to fall and a ceiling above which development was unlikely to rise. The result has been that for large segments of the population, traditional forms of social organization have remained a viable adaptation for the sharing of limited resources within families. Such an adaptation involves a paradox, however, since it is related to lower utilization of contraception and hence to increased numbers of children among the poorest part of the population.

I then went on in chapter 3 to trace changes in causes of morbidity and mortality over the past century and to indicate that in several important instances medical therapy has had an impact upon the course of death rates, especially for adults. That is to say, even in the face of continuing economic stagnation, mortality fell perceptibly so that by the time the U.S. Public Health Service assumed responsibility for Indian health care, death rates were already at a relatively low level. It was the infectious diseases and maternal mortality from sepsis that had declined. However, man-made and degenerative diseases increased both in absolute and relative importance.

The discussion of mortality patterns and the reservation economy in the first three chapters led to the following conclusions. First, there is evidence that during the first several decades of the present century, mortality rates actually increased as economic conditions deteriorated. Second, medical intervention resulted in a decline in some important causes of death beginning in the late 1940s and 1950s. Third, as these infectious diseases declined, even in the absence of significant economic improvements, accidents increased in both absolute and relative importance as a cause of mortality. Fourth, the emergence of accidents was the result of a growing use of motor vehicles and other implements by people who are especially susceptible to accidents because of their marginal position in traditional Navajo life and in the larger society. Acting-out behavior which is reflected in accidents of all sorts is not randomly distributed among Indian tribes, however, but is related to traditional patterns of social organization and social control. To the degree that economic nondevelopment encourages the persistence of these older behavior patterns even as access to motor vehicles and other implements increases, accidents will remain an important cause of mortality. Fifth, there is some evidence that the same segment of the Navajo population that has the greatest likelihood of dying from accidents—young adult men—also has the highest levels of hypertension, suggesting that in the future, morbidity and mortality patterns may continue to evolve as this cohort ages.

In chapters 4 and 5, I turned my attention to changes in Navajo health care beliefs and practices. Navajo theories of disease hold that symptomatic relief may be obtained from any number of practitioners, including physicians, while the true cause may be treated by traditional means. Thus when Anglo medical care proved effective, first in the case of surgery and then with antibiotics, increasing numbers of people made use of it without necessarily calling into question their own religious beliefs. In recent years, however, there has been a decline in the number of singers and simultaneously an increase in other religions—notably Christianity and the Native North American (peyote) Church—which also have healing aspects and are better suited to present economic and social conditions. These new conditions are related to the decline in the livestock economy which makes it increasingly difficult to sponsor long and expensive ceremonies; and to the long absences from home of many men in search of wage work, which make them unavailable for the rigorous apprenticeships that must be served in order to become singers.

Chapter 5 described patterns of utilization of Anglo medical care and how such care has changed in response to various factors including Navajos' perceptions of its efficacy. Changes in availability of beds and manpower have been important, especially from the 1930s through the 1960s. More recently, changes in the most important causes of morbidity have become significant. As the epidemic diseases have waned, utilization has become more discretionary and is related to degree of involvement in wage work and level of education. It has been argued that historically class differences in mortality have become evident as epidemics have waned because mass diseases were less likely to observe distinctions of rank than are the man-made and degenerative diseases whose etiology is explained largely by psychosocial factors (Antonovsky 1967). A roughly similar argument is made here in respect of utilization of care. As epidemic diseases wane and education increases, greater differences in patterns of health care behavior emerge, such that the more acculturated seek treatment for conditions that are not life threatening and which have only recently begun to be perceived as problems about which the health care system should do something. As in the larger society, after a threshold of acculturation is passed, cultural and social class differences in utilization may again diminish (Kunitz et al. 1975).

The mortality decline among Navajos has been different from that in the larger U.S. society in respect of both cause and duration. Medical therapy has been more significant and the decline in rate far more rapid among the former than among the latter. Even now when crude mortality rates are very similar, the proportionate contribution of different causes varies among populations. Nonetheless, in all instances infectious diseases are giving way to man-made and degenerative diseases—that is, to the new morbidities.

This shift in disease patterns has meant that the health professions and medical specialties have had to adjust to new conditions. For example, to survive the decline in infectious childhood diseases, it has been proposed that pediatrics concern itself increasingly with family, developmental, emotional, and community problems (Pless 1974). This professional imperative to survive and expand has contributed to the labeling of a variety of conditions as diseases—what some recent critics have called medicalization. But the expansionism of professions must be seen within the context of a liberal welfare state in which the amelioration of social and personal problems has often—but not always—been considered a matter of governmental concern. Moreover, the social and human services have grown rapidly not simply because there has been widespread agreement that there are many problems that require amelioration but because employment itself in service occupations has sometimes been viewed as a means of providing jobs in labor surplus areas—notably in urban and rural ghettos during the War on Poverty of the 1960s. The recruitment of workers and the creation of paraprofessions in the human services meant that a sizable number of people were taught to define a variety of conditions—such as teenage pregnancies, learning problems, and drug use—as health problems.

For all these reasons the health occupations have been increasingly involved in broadening generally accepted views of what is considered within their purview. The data in earlier chapters indicate that the same process is taking place on the Navajo reservation. Indeed, as a result of the relative rapidity of the mortality decline and the peculiar structure of the Navajos' economy, much of what has taken place in the larger society is visible in extreme form on the reservation. For example, I have said that unemployment and underemployment on the reservation is around 50 percent and that of the people who are employed, two-thirds work in the service sector. In such a situation, the few available jobs are avidly sought, and the professional ideologies of those who control or influence the employing agencies are generally accepted. Moreover, as in most such programs, those hired are the best educated and least unemployable (Goldberg 1971:16). The people who fit this category on the Navajo reservation have in the past generally been those with least stake in the traditional system, although this situation must be rapidly changing as the livestock economy becomes decreasingly viable. Nonetheless, it has been shown that Navajo paraprofessionals in the health field are more likely to share their professional supervisors' conceptions of problems than the concepts of the community they are assumed to represent (Kane and McConatha 1975).

Elsewhere I have discussed in detail how this situation works with regard to alcohol treatment programs (Levy and Kunitz 1974, 1981; Kunitz and Levy 1974). Suffice it to say here that heavy drinking, along with its sequelae of delirium tremens, blackouts, and tremulousness, was common among young Navajo men as far back in reservation history as we can determine. It was not the result only of the stress of acculturation and deprivation but was deeply embedded in Navajo life and values. Anglo professionals, however, regard it as a sign of maladaptation and as a disease to be treated, and this view is shared by the Navajos working with them. But the situation is more complicated than that, for the disease concept of alcoholism gives scientific legitimacy to the view that heavy drinking is inappropriate, as indeed it is in the world of motor vehicles, little spare cash, and obligations requiring punctuality and regular attendance at schools and jobs. For people moving into this new world, this new way of defining heavy drinking becomes a mechanism by which traditional behavior may be discredited. In this instance, then, the disease concept of alcoholism becomes a means by which a group of emerging importance may legitimize itself and confer the label of deviance on others.

This example suggests that behavior has remained constant while the explanation for it and meaning attached to it have changed. But this is only one side of the equation, for there is no doubt that there have been real changes in the health of the population and in the demand for services to which providers of services must respond. That is to say, health professionals are not only moral entrepreneurs with a license to define normal and abnormal. The examples of patterns of surgery, hospital use by the elderly, and overall changes in hospital utilization during the past fifty years illustrate this other side of the equation.

I have used variations in surgical procedures to illustrate two points. First, in comparing those of equal complexity but varying degrees of urgency I showed that the least urgent (hysterectomy) was best explained by variables that measure aspects of modernization rather than accessibility of services. This suggests that discretionary procedures are most likely to be used by people who share the values of Anglo providers of care. The comparison was meant to illustrate the larger point that to the degree that diseases change from those urgently requiring hospital treatment to those where treatment is discretionary, characteristics of patients and the determinants of utilization will change. In general, those who are most acculturated to the dominant society and who share the professionals' definitions of the conditions requiring treatment will be the ones who undergo the nonurgent procedures. The second point illustrated by the discussion of gynecological procedures is that not urgency alone but also the meaning of a procedure determines its incidence. Not only hysterectomies but all gynecological procedures are best explained by the modernization variables. This is so even in the case of Caesarean sections where urgency is likely to be greater than with the others.

Clearly one important factor is the desire to limit the number of children, but this can hardly explain the pattern of Caesarean sections and may not explain all hysterectomies. I believe that the willingness to control fertility, either surgically or with less permanent methods, may be related to women's ideas about the inevitability not only of procreation but of all the symptoms that go with it, including the pain of prolonged labor, the distress occasioned by weakened pelvic musculature after bearing many children, and dysmenorrhea. There can be no doubt that physicians, nurses, and health educators inform people that methods are available to deal with these conditions, but the degree to which their advice is accepted is largely determined by characteristics of the women and the situations in which they live.

I emphasize not only individual characteristics but the living situation as well because there is evidence that social organization is another important determinant of health care utilization. It is clearly related to contraceptive use, women living in dense kin networks being less likely to be users.

Social organization is also related to hospitalization of the elderly. Nuclear families are most prevalent where wage work is most common. Indeed, it is stable wage work that seems to make this form of family organization possible. And it is in just this setting that the elderly are most likely to be hospitalized (Gutmann 1971). The interaction with the health care system is, however, complex. There must be a place to put the elderly, which only became possible as extended care facilities were built and as the pressure on general hospitals was eased by a lessening in demand for acute care pediatric beds. But health care providers did not generally seek to make more work for themselves by defining old age as a disease. In fact, some express anger at families who do not care for their elders as they once did but instead dump them on health and social service agencies. The families that do this, however, often have little choice as they tend to be the ones whose involvement in wage work has deprived them of the necessary manpower to care for the dependent at home.

Perhaps nowhere is the controlling role of the health care system thought to be more important than in the area of hospital utilization. There is even a corollary to Parkinson's Law which says that the number of patients expands to fill the available beds. This is undoubtedly true in some instances but is clearly not universal (White et al. 1976). The data from 1933 through the 1970s support this assertion. They show that when morbidity rates were high in the 1930s, 1940s, and 1950s, opening, then closing, and then opening beds again resulted in major changes in rates of hospitalization. By the 1960s and 1970s when morbidity patterns were shifting and becoming less severe, hospitalization rates declined even as the number of beds remained constant. That the decline in number of beds per 1,000 population during these two decades was not responsible for declining hospitalization rates is suggested by the fact that occupancy rates also declined, indicating no overwhelming pressure on hospitals from an underserved clientele. Thus in the long run, major changes in disease patterns have had considerable impact on rates of hospital utilization.

Health care providers, then, react to and create needs in the populations they serve. This is not new. Fifty years ago physicians were attempting to persuade Navajos that hospital treatment was best for their most prevalent ills. Navajos remained appropriately skeptical until effective therapy was demonstrated, whereupon they sought care in increasing numbers. A similar process is at work at present but with results that are as yet uncertain. The role of medicine has been both educational and therapeutic in the not-too-distant past. Education is proceeding apace. As the examples of alcohol use, treatment of the elderly, and childbearing suggest, it helps people adapt to a changing world by providing scientific legitimacy for new ways of acting, by defining new problems, and by redefining old ones. Because, however, the conditions with which medicine must increasingly deal are largely psychosocial in origin, they are much less susceptible to therapeutic or preventive measures than, say, tuberculosis. Thus, the role of medicine as legitimate labeler of problems has increased in stature based upon therapeutic successes in the past. Its present role is made increasingly problematic, however, as the conditions it confronts—violence, problems of the elderly, population control, learning and behavioral disorders—become increasingly complex. Since many of the most serious and difficult problems—the major determinants of mortality, for instance—appear to be rooted in traditional patterns of ecological adaptation and social organization, they are likely to be especially refractory to medical intervention and will respond only to profound changes in Navajo life. To the degree that the health professions deal with these issues, they will move more and more into ambiguous regions where medical expertise may often be misapplied and even wrong in respect of the explanations it offers and treatments it recommends.

One consequence of the epidemiologic transition has been that the germ theory of disease is no longer the professionally unifying paradigm it once was. The result is increasing diversity within the profession, as new problems for which new explanations are necessary become manifest. On the one hand are those who are skeptical of medicine's past accomplishments and believe that its present and future role must involve concern with issues of the environment and individual life-style. On the other are those who believe in medicine's heroic past and the promise it implies for an equally glorious future, but only if the definition of disease is limited to problems of physiological imbalance in individuals rather than extended to include the social problems of populations (Seldin 1975, 1976).

As in the case of the germ theory in the first two-thirds of the nineteenth century (Ackerknecht 1947), one's position with regard to these issues is a political litmus test. Those on the left are likely to believe that the promise of medical cures is simply a technical fix made to divert public attention from the pathological consequences of an iniquitous social order. What is needed is basic social change which will result in better health for all.

Those on the right are more likely to believe that the left, either out of ignorance or willfulness, misrepresents the accomplishments and promise of medicine in order to further a political agenda that is not based upon careful scrutiny of objective evidence.

The material presented in this study suggests that the issue cannot be reduced to such simple positions. There can be no doubt that social institutions profoundly influence the causes and levels of mortality and morbidity. There is also no doubt that in the twentieth century specific medical measures have been significant in reducing some important causes of morbidity and mortality, even in the face of little or no social change. It is likely that as man-made and degenerative causes of mortality and morbidity are diverse in origin, some will be susceptible and others refractory to medical interventions. The truth ought not be predetermined but pursued scrupulously in each case and, as far as possible, not held hostage to politically based preconceptions.

APPENDIX I

DATA AND METHODS

In a number of places throughout this study, multiple regression is used with rates of measures of hospital utilization or mortality as the dependent variables. This appendix describes the sources of data and the types of analyses that have been used.

Several sources of data have been used: (1) hospital discharge records of Navajo patients residing on the reservation who have been seen in Indian Service and contract hospitals in the Navajo, Phoenix, and Albuquerque areas of the Indian Health Service from fiscal years 1972 through 1978; (2) population estimates of Navajos residing in the eighteen land management districts of the reservation in 1975; (3) economic data gathered in 1974 by the Survey Research Center at Brigham Young University; and (4) death certificates from the Navajo area from 1972 to 1978. I shall describe each briefly in turn.

The hospital records consist of discharge sheets which have been computerized and include age, sex, tribe, community of residence, primary, secondary, and tertiary diagnoses, types of surgical procedures done, dates of admission and discharge, and some additional information. Because the IHS is the major provider of health care to Navajos on the reservation, and because most of the care not provided directly is paid for by contract funds, reporting of hospitalizations is virtually complete. The one important exception appears to be workmen's compensation cases which are often cared for in non-IHS facilities and paid for by a third party that does not report to the Indian Health Service. In the present instance, the loss of cases is thought to be minimal.

Unfortunately, these records do not include such information as marital status, parity, occupation, and income.

Population estimates for land management districts are based upon tribal enrollment data and school censuses for 1975 and include only total population and no information on age structure. Methods of estimation are described in detail elsewhere (Davis and Kunitz 1978). It must be pointed out that Navajo population has been notoriously difficult to estimate and enumerate. There is good reason to believe that the U.S. Census has consistently undercounted Navajos, some estimates suggest by as much as 20 or 25 percent. By contrast, the Bureau of Indian Affairs population register is known to have overestimated the population (U.S. Bureau of the Census 1977). The figures I have used are based upon estimates made by the Navajo Tribe's Office of Information and Statistics in consultation with the BIA and the Census Bureau (Faich 1976). When these are projected from 1975 to 1980 (by adding births and subtracting deaths), the result is a reservation population upwards of 148,000. Preliminary analyses of the 1980 U.S. Census gives a figure of about 128,000, approximately 14 percent less.

In order to calculate hospitalization and mortality rates, the 1975 estimate of land management district populations has been used. In calculating age-specific rates of certain causes of mortality in chapter 3, a 1978 estimation of age and sex structure of the population based upon the 1975 figures has been used. In each case it must be kept in mind that the denominator (population size) may be as much as 15 percent overestimated. Thus, the rates I have estimated may be as much as 15 percent lower than they are in reality. In point of fact, the difference is likely to be less than 15 percent as the census enumeration is still probably somewhat low despite major efforts at improving its accuracy.

The 1974 economic survey used land management districts as sampling frames. Considering the difficulties described above in enumerating the population, developing an adequate sampling frame would be a formidable task indeed. Undoubtedly there are inaccuracies in the survey. Nonetheless, it is the only one available in recent years that gathered comparable data from all areas of the reservation and as such is of considerable value. Except for average distance to the nearest hospital providing surgery or simply general services, the independent variables are drawn from this source. They are displayed in table 2.9 (chapter 2).

The 1974 economic survey (Wistisen et al. 1975) collected data on a very large number of variables, only a few of which have been used in the present study. Those chosen reflect socioeconomic characteristics of the populations in different land management districts (median family and per capita income, proportion of income from wages and welfare, proportions of men and women working full-time, average educational level); housing conditions that might influence health status (proportion of families with a bathroom and proportion living in hogans); and population structure (average household size, average age of male and female household heads). Proportion of families owning a motor vehicle was included because of the importance of automobile accidents in contributing to both mortality and morbidity rates. The relationships among them are displayed in the biplot in figure 2.4.

When a larger set of variables was examined by correlation analysis, strong relationships were found which indicated that many variables might be safely ignored. For example, the correlation coefficients between proportion of households having a bathroom and proportion with indoor plumbing was 0.89; with proportion of families hauling water 0.87; with proportion having electricity 0.80; and with proportion having a telephone 0.70.

The two independent variables that do not appear in the economic survey are average distance from the nearest general hospital and average distance from the nearest hospital providing surgery. These were calculated in the following way. Each land management district is comprised of several smaller administrative and governmental units called chapters. Population size of each chapter is known, although no other economic or demographic data were available at this level of analysis. (The 1980 census when it becomes available will treat chapters as enumeration districts, making possible much more detailed analyses.) The shortest distance by road from each community where a chapter house was located to the nearest general hospital and nearest hospital providing surgery were calculated using a road map of the reservation. A weighted average distance for each land management district was then calculated.

Mortality data come from death certificates sent by each state to the National Center for Vital Statistics for processing. Any certificate listing the dead individual as an American Indian is put on a computer tape and sent to the Indian Health Service. Tribal membership is not known, simply whether the individual was an American Indian. Tribal membership is inferred by place of residence. For example, an American Indian whose residence was a Navajo reservation community would be assumed to have been a Navajo. Indians of other tribes do live on the Navajo reservation, either because they work for a government agency or are married to Navajos, and this introduces an unknown but small amount of error.

Community of residence is coded on each certificate. In order to protect privacy as well as to make the data compatible with other sources we have used, communities were aggregated into land management districts. Unfortunately, because the Utah part of the reservation is so sparsely settled, county of residence rather than community of residence is coded (in this case San Juan County). The county includes a small number of Utes and Paiutes, and from the certificates there is no way of distinguishing between them and Navajos. Because the number of deaths was small, I allocated them all to those Navajo reservation land management districts located at least partially in San Juan County. The proportionate distribution of deaths was based upon a count of dwelling units in that part of each of the relevant districts (2, 8, 9, and 12) as determined from a detailed BIA road map of the reservation (BIA Federal-Aid Indian Road System, Navajo Area, 1974). Once the number of dwellings in the Utah portion of each district was known, the proportionate distribution could be calculated and deaths randomly assigned in the proper proportion. Undoubtedly this procedure introduced some error, but the number of deaths involved was small (233 out of a total of 6,747 from 1972–1978) and the distortion introduced was not thought to be great.

Regression analysis is employed to explain the observed rates of the dependent variables. In each case the dependent variable is an average annual ratio for the period 1972–1976. This time span was selected for two reasons: (1) in order to use 1974, for which the socioeconomic data were available, as a midpoint; and (2) because in July, 1977 the Winslow IHS hospital was closed, thus changing the access to care for populations in those land management districts previously served by that facility.

The regression employed is the stepwise procedure with maximum R^2 improvement (MAXR). This technique is considered superior to a simple stepwise procedure because it does not settle on a single model. MAXR begins by finding the one-variable model producing the highest R^2. Then, another variable expected to yield the greatest increase in R^2 is added. Once the two-variable model is obtained, the variable in the model is compared to all those not in the model, and MAXR considers the improvement in the R^2 that each potential switch offers. The difference between the stepwise technique and the maximum R^2 improvement method is that MAXR evaluates all possibilities before a final choice is made.

Multiple regression allows us to consider one dependent variable at a time. For that reason, some do not regard it as a true multivariate technique. The biplot, by contrast, is a multivariate technique, as it permits the analysis of the relationships between a number of variables. Described in detail in chapter 1, the biplot is used several times in subsequent chapters to display graphically the relationship between variables and land management districts. In each instance in which the biplot is used, as in each use of multiple regression, the analyses are performed at the ecological level. That is, characteristics of land management district populations (or entire tribes in chapter 1) are the units of analysis, not characteristics of individuals taken one at a time.

Ecological analyses pose problems, for one runs the risk of committing what has been called the "ecological fallacy," making mistaken inferences about individuals based upon the characteristics of the group to which they belong (Robinson 1950; Duncan and Davis 1953; Goodman 1953, 1959; Iverson 1973). An example of such an error would be the following: In chapters 3 and 5, I have shown that gynecological surgery rates are high among populations where a high proportion of income is derived from wage work, where educational levels are high, and where family organization is likely to be nuclear. I have inferred that it is women who have these characteristics and live in these families who have the high rates of surgery. But that might be a mistake. The women who have the surgery may in fact be poorly educated, not dependent upon wage work, and live in other kinds of families. Without gathering individual-level data, one cannot be certain that one has avoided or committed the ecological fallacy.

There are several points to be made about this. First, quite apart from making inferences about individuals, it is worth knowing that highly acculturated populations have high rates of gynecological surgery, even if on further investigation it turns out to be the relatively few unacculturated women in that generally acculturated population who account for the high rates (Menzel 1950). Second, one is not always making inferences about individual correlations. A high correlation between low infant mortality rates and high physician/population ratios does not refer to the same individuals or assume that doctors are infants, or vice versa (Menzel 1950). Third, just because it is possible to commit the ecological fallacy does not mean that an error is made each time one does an ecological correlation. It is at least as likely that one will make a reasonable and even correct inference as a mistake. Fourth, in principle the issue is broader than simply moving from aggregate data to inferences about individuals. The same problem exists moving from any level of analysis to another, for instance when making inferences about counties from state data. As Blalock (1964:98) has observed, it would be upsetting if the fundamental nature of the relationship between variables changed as levels of analysis shifted. What does happen is that the manner in which outside and possibly disturbing variables influence the dependent and independent variables changes (Blalock 1964:95–114).

Nonetheless, a potentially real problem of making wrong inferences does exist, and it is appropriate to keep that in mind. Though many of my interpretations are expressed assertively, I believe that the inferences I have drawn about individuals, while entirely plausible and most probably correct, should be the basis for developing hypotheses to be tested by field research. Having said that, however, it is also important to remember that much useful information about population aggregates is to be derived from the ecological analyses, whether or not the reader accepts the inferences about individual behavior based upon them.

APPENDIX II

TABLE 1

MORTALITY RATES FOR SELECTED CAUSES, U.S. POPULATION, 1900–1970
(per 100,000 population)

Year	Respiratory tuberculosis	Influenza/ pneumonia	Gastro- enteritis	Cirrhosis	Suicide	Motor vehicle accidents	Falls	All others
1900	194.4	202.2	142.7	12.5	10.2	—	—	72.3
1910	153.8	155.9	115.4	13.3	15.3	1.8	15.4	67.0
1920	113.1	207.3	53.7	7.1	10.2	10.3	11.8	47.9
1930	71.1	102.5	26.0	7.2	15.6	26.7	14.7	38.4
1940	45.9	70.3	10.3	8.6	14.4	26.2	17.2	29.8
1950	22.5	31.3	5.1	9.2	11.4	23.1	13.8	23.7
1960	6.1	37.3	4.4	11.3	10.6	21.3	10.6	20.4
1970	2.6	30.9	0.6	15.5	11.6	26.9	8.3	21.2

Source: Bureau of the Census, *Historical Statistics of the U.S., Colonial Times to 1970, Bicentennial edition*, pt. 1, Washington, D.C.: U.S. Government Printing Office, 1975, p. 58.

TABLE 2
RESPIRATORY TUBERCULOSIS MORTALITY RATE PER 100,000, MASSACHUSETTS, 1861–1970

Year	Rate
1861	365.2
1870	343.3
1880	308.1
1890	258.6
1900	196.3
1910	138.3
1920	96.8
1930	57.2
1940	34.6
1950	9.3
1960	6.0
1970	2.4

Source: Bureau of the Census, *Historical Statistics of the United States, Colonial Times to 1970, Bicentennial edition*, pt. 1. Washington, D.C.: U.S. Government Printing Office, 1975, p. 63.

TABLE 3
HOSPITAL UTILIZATION, U.S. POPULATION, 1931–1970

Year	General and special hospitals Admissions/ 1,000 population	Average length of stay	Tuberculosis hospitals Admissions/ 1,000 population	Average length of stay
1931	56	15.3	0.6	254
1935	59	15.0	0.7	257
1940	74	13.7	0.7	269
1945	120	16.5	0.7	253
1950	110	10.6	0.7	233
1955	125	9.9	0.7	219
1960	136	9.3	0.4	200
1965	146	9.1	0.3	183
1970	152	9.5	0.2	122

Source: Bureau of the Census, *Historical Statistics of the U.S., Colonial Times to 1970, Bicentennial edition*, pt. 1. Washington, D.C.: U.S. Government Printing Office, 1975. p. 82.

Notes

1. MORTALITY, FERTILITY, AND SOCIAL ORGANIZATION

1. The biplot is a graphical display based upon the singular value decomposition of a data matrix. For an $n \times m$ matrix Y of rank r, the singular value decomposition of Y is

$$Y = \sum_{i=1}^{r} \lambda_i p_i q'_\alpha \qquad (1)$$

The p_α and q'_α (column vectors) corresponding to the α-th singular value are referred to as the α-th singular column and singular row, respectively. The biplot displays the rank z approximation obtained by truncating equation (1) after two terms. $\lambda_i^{\frac{1}{2}}$ is the α-th singular value (eigenvalue) of Y.

The ratio $\lambda_i/\Sigma\lambda_i$ is a measure of the adequacy of the biplot as an approximation. For the 10×8 data matrix of table 1.2, the following results are obtained.

α	$\lambda_i^{\frac{1}{2}}$	λ_i	$(\lambda_i/\Sigma\lambda_i) \times 100$
1	6.373	40.62	50.77
2	4.558	20.77	25.96
3	3.305	10.92	13.65
4	2.181	4.76	5.94
Residual	–	2.93	3.66
Total		80.00	100.00

The first two singular values account for 77% of the total variability in table 1.2, suggesting that the biplot is a reasonable approximation.

The mathematical details and examples of the biplot may be found in Gabriel et al. (1974) and Gabriel (1971).

2. ECONOMIC AND DEMOGRAPHIC CHANGE

1. In a personal communication, David Aberle has pointed out that it is a common error to assume that people without livestock permits do not raise stock. His data from several parts of the reservation indicate that many people without permits do raise stock. Data from the Lake Powell Research Project collected on the western end of the reservation indicate that no one, even those with permits, can survive on livestock alone, though it may make a substantial contribution to the support of some families.

3. DISEASE PATTERNS

1. The table below displays data on in-patients in all Navajo and the one Hopi hospital for the years 1916–1917 and 1919–1920. Several noteworthy points emerge. First, in 1916–1917 there was no significant difference in death rates among any of the hospitals. If, however, the data are disaggregated and deaths among sanatorium patients are compared with deaths among other patients, then a significant difference does become obvious ($X^2 = 33.86$, d.f. = 5, $p<.0001$). Not surprisingly, tuberculosis patients had higher death rates than other patients in a nonepidemic period.

Second, during the pandemic in 1919–1920 (when unfortunately deaths cannot be disaggregated for sanatorium patients), there was a significant increase in mortality among patients in the Hopi, San Juan, and Navajo hospitals

HOSPITAL ADMISSIONS AND DEATHS, 1916–1920

	1916–17		1919–20		Comparison, 1916–1917 + 1919–1920		
	Discharged alive	Died	Discharged alive	Died	X^2	df	p
Leupp	146	3	188	2	N.S.		
Moqui	437	7	296	16	9.08	1	< .01
Navajo:							
school	710	10					
sanatorium	71	7					
total	782	17	1,121	95	31.16	1	< .001
Western Navajo	245	2	230	0	N.S.		
San Juan:							
school	228	1					
hospital	152	0					
total	380	1	757	20	9.02	1	< .01
TOTAL	1,989	30	2,592	133			
Comparison:							
X^2	7.17		49.2				
df	4		4				
p	> .05		< .001				

Source: Annual Reports, Commissioner of Indian Affairs

(for a description, see Reagan 1919). The increase was most impressive in the Navajo hospital where the sanatorium was located, suggesting that tuberculosis patients may have been much more susceptible than others. There was no increase in the Western Navajo or Leupp hospitals, indicating either that the pandemic did not have as much impact in the less densely settled areas as it did elsewhere, or that people simply died before ever getting to a hospital.

2. This estimate is higher than any of those reported in the 1974 economic survey (Wistisen et al. 1975, I: 93), which showed that the highest proportion of homes having indoor plumbing was 49 percent in district 9. The correlation between proportion of homes having a bathroom and proportion having indoor plumbing is 0.89 (see appendix I).

3. I have not discussed diabetes in this chapter. It has often been observed to be of high prevalence among Navajos and other American Indians, and conventional wisdom has it that Indians do not suffer complications as non-Indians do. Clinicians on the Navajo reservation are now beginning to observe, however, that all the sequelae found among non-Indians are becoming increasingly frequent among Navajos, notably vascular complications. As yet these are clinical impressions unsupported by epidemiological studies. It is of considerable interest that renal dialysis units have been installed in a number of Navajo Area hospitals to treat patients, most of whom have kidney damage secondary to their diabetic vascular disease. It is symbolically appropriate that in the new Tuba City hospital, this unit is in what had originally been planned as a pediatric ward.

5. HEALTH CARE UTILIZATION

1. One of the consequences of transfer was the rebirth of the "anthropological approach" as contracts were written with several universities to develop research and demonstration projects. The University of North Carolina, the University of California at Berkeley, and Cornell University Medical College all had contracts. The Cornell-Many Farms Project was the best known (Adair and Deuschle 1970). Though much useful data was produced, it is doubtful that any innovations resulting from the projects had a lasting impact on the provision of health care, for reasons discussed by Adair and Deuschle (1970; see also Kane and Kane 1970).

2. Recall that these data pertain to the period before the Winslow Hospital was closed.

References

Aberle, D. F.
    1963   Some sources of flexibility in Navajo social organization. *Southwestern Journal of Anthropology* 19:1–8.
    1966   *The Peyote Religion Among the Navajo.* Chicago: Aldine Publishing Company.
    1969   A plan for Navajo economic development. *Toward Economic Development for Native American Communities.* A compendium of papers submitted to the Sub-Committee on Economy in Government of the Joint Economic Committee of the Congress of the U.S. Washington, D.C.: U.S. Government Printing Office.
    1981   A century of Navajo kinship change. *Canadian Journal of Anthropology* 2:21–36.
    1982   The future of Navajo religion. In *Navajo Religion and Culture: Selected Views.* Papers in Honor of Leland C. Wyman. Ed. D. M. Brugge and C. J. Frisbie. Santa Fe: Museum of New Mexico Press.

Ackerknecht, E. H.
    1948   Anti-contagionism between 1821 and 1867. *Bulletin of the History of Medicine* 22: 562–593.

Adair, J., and K. W. Deuschle
    1970   *The People's Health.* New York: Appleton-Century-Crofts.

Alfred, B.
    1970   Blood pressure changes among male Navaho migrants to an urban environment. *Canadian Review of Sociology and Anthropology* 7: 189–200.

Antonovsky, A.
    1967   Social class, life expectancy and overall mortality. *Milbank Memorial Fund Quarterly* 45:31–73.

Aronson, J. D.
    1948   Protective vaccination against tuberculosis with special reference to BCG vaccination. *American Review of Tuberculosis* 58:255–281.

Aronson, J. D., and C. E. Palmer
    1946   Experience with BCG vaccine in the control of tuberculosis among North American Indians. *Public Health Reports* 61:802–820.

Aronson, J. D., C. E. Aronson, and H. C. Taylor
  1958   A twenty-year appraisal of BCG vaccination in the control of tuber-
         culosis. *Archives of Internal Medicine* 101:881–893.
Bailey, F. L.
  1950   *Some Sex Beliefs and Practices in a Navajo Community.* Cambridge,
         Mass.: Peabody Museum, Harvard University.
Berggren, W. L., D. C. Ewbank, and G. G. Berggren
  1981   Reduction of mortality in rural Haiti through a primary health-
         care program. *New England Journal of Medicine* 304:1324–1330.
Black, F. L.
  1966   Measles endemicity in insular populations: critical community size
         and its evolutionary implication. *Journal of Theoretical Biology* 11:
         207–211.
  1975   Infectious diseases in primitive societies. *Science* 187:515–518.
Blalock, H. M., Jr.
  1964   *Causal Inferences in Nonexperimental Research.* Chapel Hill: The Uni-
         versity of North Carolina Press.
Bollinger, C. C., W. C. Carrier, and W. J. Ledger
  1970   Intrauterine contraception in Indians of the American Southwest.
         American Journal of Obstetrics and Gynecology 106:669–675.
Bombardier, C., V. R. Fuchs, L. A. Lillard, and K. E. Warner
  1977   Socioeconomic factors affecting the utilization of surgical opera-
         tions. *New England Journal of Medicine* 297:669–705.
Boyce, G. A.
  1974   *When Navajos Had Too Many Sheep: The 1940s.* San Francisco:
         Indian Historian Press.
Brenner, C., K. S. Reisinger, and K. D. Rogers
  1974   Navajo infant mortality, 1970. *Public Health Reports* 89:353–359.
Brewer, I. W.
  1906   Tuberculosis among the Indians of Arizona and New Mexico. *New
         York State Medical Journal* 84:981–983.
Brown, R. C., B. S. Gurunanjapa, R. J. Hawk, and D. Bitsuie
  1970   The epidemiology of accidents among the Navajo Indians. *Public
         Health Reports* 85:881–888.
Brugge, D.
  1972   *Historic Use and Occupancy of the Tuba City-Moencopi Area.* Revised
         and edited by J. L. Correll. Window Rock, Arizona: The Research
         Section, The Navajo Tribe.
Buikstra, J. E., ed.
  1981   *Prehistoric Tuberculosis in the Americas.* Scientific paper no. 5. Evan-
         ston, Illinois: Northwestern University Archeological Program.
Callaway, D. G.
  in press   *The Impact of Industrialization on Navajo Household Organization.*
             Bulletin 51, Lake Powell Research Project. Los Angeles: Institute
             of Geophysics, University of California.
Callaway, D. G., J. E. Levy, and E. B. Henderson
  1976   *The Effects of Power Production and Strip Mining on Local Navajo*

Populations. Bulletin 22, Lake Powell Research Project. Los Angeles: Institute of Geophysics, University of California.

Campbell, J.
1970 *The Masks of God: Primitive Mythology.* New York: Viking (Compass, ed.) [1st edition, 1959].

Carr, B. A., and E. S. Lee
1978 Navajo tribal mortality: a life table analysis of the leading causes of death. *Social Biology* 25:279–287.

Cassel, J.
1970 Physical illness in response to stress. In *Social Stress*, ed. S. Levine and N. A. Scotch. Chicago: Aldine Publishing Company.
1974 Psychosocial processes and "stress": theoretical formulation. *International Journal of Health Services* 4:471–482.

Cockburn, T. A.
1963 *The Evolution and Eradication of Infectious Diseases.* Baltimore: The Johns Hopkins University Press.

Cohen, B. M.
1953 Arterial hypertension among Indians of the Southwestern United States. *American Journal of Medical Sciences* 225:505–513.

Collier, J.
1933 Indian Health. *Proceedings of the Conference of State and Provincial Health Authorities of North America* 48:56–62.

Comess, L. J., P. H. Bennett, and T. A. Burch
1967 Clinical gallbladder disease in Pima Indians: its high prevalence in contrast to Framingham, Massachusetts. *New England Journal of Medicine* 277:894–898.

Commissioner of Indian Affairs
1900–1950 Annual Reports. Washington, D.C.: U.S. Government Printing Office.

Committee on Interior and Insular Affairs
1974 *Indian Health Care Improvement Act: Report of the Committee, together with additional views to accompany S. 2938.* Washington, D.C.: U.S. Government Printing Office.

Coulehan, J., S. Grant, K. Reisinger, P. Killian, K. Rogers, and C. Kaltenbach
1980 Acute rheumatic fever and rheumatic heart disease on the Navajo reservation, 1962–77. *Public Health Reports* 95:62–68.

Darby, W. J., C. G. Salsbury, W. J. McGanity, H. F. Johnson, E. B. Bridgeforth, and H. R. Sandstead
1956 A study of the dietary background and nutrition of the Navajo Indian. *Journal of Nutrition* 60 (supplement): 3–85.

Davis, S., and S. J. Kunitz
1978 Hospital utilization and elective surgery on the Navajo Indian reservation. *Social Science and Medicine* 12B:263–272.

DeJong, G.
1972 Patterns of human fertility and mortality. In *The Structure of Human Populations*, ed. G. A. Harrison and A. J. Boyce. New York: Oxford University Press.

DeStefano, F., L. Coulehan, and M. K. Wiant
   1979   Blood pressure survey on the Navajo Indian reservation. *American Journal of Epidemiology* 109:335–345.
Deuschle, K. W.
   1959   Tuberculosis among the Navajo. *American Review of Respiratory Diseases* 80:200–206.
Dobyns, H. F.
   1966   Estimating aboriginal American population, an appraisal of techniques with a new hemispheric estimate. *Current Anthropology* 7: 395–416.
   1976   *Native American Historical Demography, a Critical Bibliography.* Bloomington: Indiana University Press.
Doran, C. M.
   1972   Attitudes of 30 American Indian women towards birth control. *HSMHA Health Reports* 87:658–663.
DuBois, J.
   1978   Navajos Are Coming to Jesus. *Navajo Times*, July 27:B8–9.
Dubos, R.
   1965   *Man Adapting.* New Haven: Yale University Press.
Duncan, O. D., and B. Davis
   1953   An alternative to ecological correlation. *American Sociological Review* 18:665–666.
Elmore, H.
   1944   *Ethnobotany of the Navajo.* Albuquerque: University of New Mexico Press.
Faich, R.
   1976   Evidence in support of more revenue sharing money for the Navajo Tribe. Unpublished report. Window Rock, Arizona: Navajo Nation/Navajo Research and Statistics Center, The Navajo Tribe.
   1977   *A reapportion plan for the Navajo Tribal Council.* Window Rock, Arizona: Research and Statistics Division, Office of Program Development, The Navajo Tribe.
   1978   *Population Estimates.* Window Rock, Arizona: Information Services Department, The Navajo Tribe.
Foard, F. T.
   1950   The federal government and American Indians' health. *Journal of the American Medical Association* 142:328–331.
Fulmer, H. S. and R. W. Roberts
   1963   Coronary heart disease among the Navajo Indians. *Annals of Internal Medicine* 59:740–764.
Gabriel, K. R.
   1971   The biplot—graphic display of matrices with application in principal component analysis. *Biometrika* 58:453–467.
   1973   Canonical decomposition and biplots: notes, examples and computer program CANDEC. Jerusalem: Department of Statistics, The Hebrew University.

Gabriel, K. R., M. Hill, and N. Law-Yone
   1974   A multivariate statistical method for regionalization. *Journal of Regional Sciences* 14:89–106.
Gilbert, J.
   1955   Absence of coronary thrombosis in Navajo Indians. *California Medicine* 82:114–115.
Glenn, T.
   1976   *The Structure of Employment in the Navajo Nation, An Analysis of the Navajo Economy.* Window Rock, Arizona: Office of Program Development, The Navajo Tribe.
Goldberg, G. S.
   1971   Nonprofessionals in human services. In *Nonprofessionals in the Human Services,* ed. C. Grosser, W. E. Henry, and J. G. Kelly. San Francisco: Jossey-Bass.
Goodman, L. A.
   1953   Ecological regression and behavior of individuals. *American Sociological Review* 18:663–664.
   1959   Some alternatives to ecological correlation. *American Journal of Sociology* 64:610–625.
Gregg, E. D.
   1965   *The Indians and the Nurse.* Norman: University of Oklahoma Press.
Guillemin, J.
   1980   Federal policies and Indian politics. *Transaction* May/June: 29–34.
Gutmann, D.
   1971   Dependency, illness, and survival among Navajo men. In *Prediction of Life Span,* ed. E. Palmore. Lexington, Mass.: D.C. Heath.
Habakkuk, H. J.
   1971   *Population Growth and Economic Development Since 1750.* Leicester: Leicester University Press.
Hadley, J. N.
   1955   Health conditions among Navajo Indians. *Public Health Reports* 70:831–836.
Haile, B.
   1937   Prostitution and Moth Way: Text and Translation. Museum of Northern Arizona, Manuscript Collection 63:11. Flagstaff.
   1950   *Legend of the Ghostway Ritual in the Male Branch of Shootingway and Sucking Way in its Legend and Practice.* St. Michaels, Ariz.: St. Michaels Press.
Haynes, S. G., M. Feinleib, and W. B. Kannel
   1980   III. Eight-year incidence of coronary heart disease. *American Journal of Epidemiology* 111:37–58.
Haynes, S. G., S. Levine, N. Scotch, M. Feinleib, and W. B. Kannel
   1978a   The relationship of psychosocial factors to coronary heart disease in the Framingham study, I. Methods and risk factors. *American Journal of Epidemiology* 107:362–383.
   1978b   II. Prevalence of coronary heart disease. *American Journal of Epidemiology* 107:384–402.

Henderson, E. B.
  1982 Kaibeto Plateau ceremonialists: 1860–1980. In *Navajo Religion and Culture: Selected Views*. Papers in honor of L. C. Wyman, ed. D. M. Brugge and C. J. Frisbie. Santa Fe: Museum of New Mexico Press.
Henderson, E. B., and J. E. Levy
  1975 *Survey of Navajo Community Studies, 1936–1974*. Bulletin 6, Lake Powell Research Project. Los Angeles: Institute of Geophysics, University of California.
Hesse, F. G.
  1964 Incidence of disease in the Navajo Indian. *Archives of Pathology* 77:553–557.
Hester, J. J.
  1962 *Early Navajo Migrations and Acculturation in the Southwest*. Papers in Anthropology no. 6. Santa Fe: Museum of New Mexico.
Hill, W. W.
  1935 The status of the hermaphrodite and transvestite in Navajo culture. *American Anthropologist* 37:273–279.
Hrdlicka, A.
  1909 *Tuberculosis among Certain Tribes of the United States*. Bulletin 42. Bureau of American Ethnology. Washington, D.C.: U.S. Government Printing Office.
Iversen, G. R.
  1973 Recovering individual data in the presence of group and individual effects. *American Journal of Sociology* 79:420–434.
James, C. D., III, and A. J. Lindsay, Jr.
  1973 Ethnoarchaeological research at Canyon del Muerto, Arizona: a Navajo example. *Ethnohistory* 20:361–374.
Johansson, S. R., and S. H. Preston
  1978 Tribal demography: the Hopi and Navajo populations as seen through manuscripts from the 1900 U.S. census. *Social Science History* 3:1–33.
Johnston, D. F.
  1966a *An Analysis of Sources of Information on the Population of the Navajo*. Bulletin 197, Bureau of American Ethnology. Washington, D.C.: U.S. Government Printing Office.
  1966b Trends in Navajo Population and Education. In *The Peyote Religion among the Navajo*, D. F. Aberle. Chicago: Aldine Publishing Co.
Jorgensen, J. G.
  1971 Indians and the metropolis. In *The American Indian in Urban Society*, ed. J. O. Waddell and O. M. Watson. Boston: Little, Brown, and Co.
Joslin, E. P.
  1940 The universality of diabetes. *Journal of the American Medical Association* 115:2033–2038.
Kaltenbach, C.
  1976 *Health Problems of the Navajo Area and Suggested Interventions*. Window Rock, Arizona: Navajo Health Authority.

Kane, R. L., and R. A. Kane
    1972   *Federal Health Care (With Reservations)!* New York: Springer Publishing Company, Inc.

Kane, R. L., and P. D. McConatha
    1975   The men in the middle: a dilemma of minority health workers. *Medical Care* 13:736–743.

Kaplan, B., and D. Johnson
    1964   The social meaning of Navajo psychopathology. In *Magic, Faith and Healing*, ed. A. Kiev. New York: Free Press of Glencoe.

Katz, P. S., and P. A. May
    1979   *Motor Vehicle Accidents on the Navajo Reservation, 1973–1975.* Window Rock, Arizona: Navajo Health Authority.

Kelly, L. C.
    1968   *The Navajo Indians and Federal Indian Policy.* Tucson: University of Arizona Press.

Kemrer, M. F.
    1974   The dynamics of western Navajo settlement, A.D. 1750–1900: An archaeological and dendrochronological analysis. Ph.D. dissertation, Department of Anthropology, University of Arizona, Tucson, Arizona.

Kessner, D. M.
    1968   *Infant, Perinatal, Maternal and Childhood Mortality in the United States.* Cambridge, Mass.: Harvard University Press.

Khattab, H.
    1974   Current Roles of Ramah Navajo Women and their Natality Behavior. Ph.D. dissertation, Department of Anthropology, University of North Carolina, Chapel Hill.

Kimball, S. T.
    1940   Navajo Population Analysis. *Navajo Medical News* 7:2–3.
    1965   Research and Concept Formation in Community Study. In *Culture and Community*, C. M. Arensberg and S. T. Kimball, New York: Harcourt, Brace and World, Inc.

Kluckhohn, C.
    1962   *Navajo Witchcraft*, 2d edition. Boston: Beacon Press.

Kluckhohn, C., and D. C. Leighton
    1946   *The Navajo.* Cambridge, Mass.: Harvard University Press.

Kositchek, R. J., M. Wurn, and R. Straus
    1961   Biochemical studies in full blooded Navajo Indians, II. Lipids and lipoproteins. *Circulation* 23:219–224.

Krug, J. A.
    1948   *The Navajo, a Long-Range Program for Navajo Rehabilitation.* Washington, D.C.: Bureau of Indian Affairs, Dept. of the Interior.

Kunitz, S. J.
    1971   The social philosophy of John Collier. *Ethnohistory* 18:213–229.
    1974a Factors influencing recent Navajo and Hopi population change. *Human Organization* 33:7–16.
    1974b Navajo and Hopi fertility, 1971–1972. *Human Biology* 46:

435–451.

1976a *The Relationship of Economic Variations to Mortality and Fertility Patterns on the Navajo Reservation.* Bulletin 20, Lake Powell Research Project. Los Angeles: Institute of Geophysics, University of California.

1976b *A Survey of Fertility Histories and Contraceptive Use Among a Group of Navajo Women.* Bulletin 21, Lake Powell Research Project. Los Angeles: Institute of Geophysics, University of California.

1977 Underdevelopment and social services on the Navajo reservation. *Human Organization* 36:398–404.

in press Speculations on the European mortality decline. *Economic History Review.*

Kunitz, S. J., and J. E. Levy

1974 Changing ideas of alcohol use among Navajo Indians. *Quarterly Journal of Studies on Alcohol* 35:243–259.

Kunitz, S. J., J. E. Levy, C. L. Odoroff, and J. Bollinger

1971 The epidemiology of alcoholic cirrhosis in two Southwestern Indian tribes. *Quarterly Journal of Studies on Alcohol* 32:706–720.

Kunitz, S. J., and J. C. Slocomb

1976 The use of surgery to avoid childbearing among Navajo and Hopi Indians. *Human Biology* 48:9–21.

Kunitz, S. J., A. A. Sorensen, and S. Cashman

1975 Changing health care opinions in Regionville. *Medical Care* 13: 549–561.

Kunitz, S. J., and M. Tsianco

1981 Kinship dependence and contraceptive use in sample of Navajo women. *Human Biology* 53:439–452.

LaBarre, W.

1938 *The Peyote Colt.* Yale University Publications in Anthropology 19. New Haven.

Lam, R. C.

1954 Gallbladder diseases among the American Indians. *The Journal-Lancet* 74:305–309.

Lamphere, L.

1979 Traditional pastoral economy. In *Economic Development in American Indian Reservations.* Native American Studies, Development Series no. 1. Albuquerque: University of New Mexico.

Landar, H.

1967 The language of pain in Navajo culture. In *Studies in Southwestern Linguistics: Meaning and History in the Languages of the American Southwest,* ed. D. Hymes and W. E. Bittle. The Hague: Mouton and Company.

Lee, R. B.

1972 Population growth and the beginnings of sedentary life among the Kung Bushmen. In *Population Growth: Anthropological Implications,* ed. B. Spooner. Cambridge, Mass.: MIT Press.

Leighton, A. H., and D. A. Kennedy

1957 Pilot study of cultural items in medical diagnosis: a field report. Mimeo.

Leighton, A. H., and D. C. Leighton
 1944 *The Navajo Door: An Introduction to Navajo Life*. Cambridge, Mass.: Harvard University Press.
Leighton, D. C., and C. Kluckhohn
 1948 *Children of the People*. Cambridge, Mass.: Harvard University Press.
Lerner, M., and O. W. Anderson
 1963 *Health Progress in the United States: 1900–1960*. Chicago: University of Chicago Press.
Levy, J. E.
 1962*a* Some trends in Navajo health behavior. Window Rock, Arizona: U.S. Public Health Service, Division of Indian Health. Mimeo.
 1962*b* Medical decision making in a Navajo outfit: preliminary report. Tuba City, Arizona: U.S. Public Health Service Indian Hospital. Mimeo.
 1964*a* The fate of Navajo twins. *American Anthropologist* 66:883–887.
 1964*b* Interpreter training program. Window Rock, Arizona: U.S. Public Health Service, Division of Indian Health. Mimeo.
 1965 Navajo suicide. *Human Organization* 24:308–318.
 1980 Who benefits from energy resource development: the special case of the Navajo Indians. *The Social Science Journal* 17:1–19.
 in press *Hand Trembling, Frenzy Witchcraft and Moth Madness: A Study of Navajo Seizure Disorders*. Tucson: University of Arizona Press.
Levy, J. E., and S. J. Kunitz
 1971 Indian reservations, anomie, and social pathologies. *Southwestern Journal of Anthropology* 27:97–128.
 1974 *Indian Drinking: Navajo Practices and Anglo-American Theories*. New York: John Wiley and Sons, Inc.
 1981 Economic and political factors inhibiting the use of basic research findings in Indian alcoholism programs. *Journal of Studies on Alcohol*, Supplement 9:60–72.
Levy, J. E., S. J. Kunitz, and M. Everett
 1969 Navajo criminal homicide. *Southwestern Journal of Anthropology* 25:124–152.
Levy, J. E., R. Neutra, and D. Parker
 1977 Life careers of Navajo epileptics. *Social Science and Medicine* 13B:53–66.
Lockett, C.
 1939 Midwives and childbirth among the Navajo. *Plateau* 12:15–17.
Loughlin, B. W.
 1962 A study of the needs of the pregnant women in a selected group of Navajo women. M.P.H. thesis, School of Public Health, University of North Carolina, Chapel Hill.
Lower, G. M., Jr., and M. S. Kanarek
 1982 The mutation theory of chronic, noninfectious disease: relevance to epidemiologic theory. *American Journal of Epidemiology* 115:803–817.
Luckert, K. W.
 1975 *The Navajo Hunter Tradition*. Tucson: University of Arizona Press.

Lyon, J. P.
1978   *The Indian Elder, A Forgotten American.* Albuquerque: National Indian Council on Aging.
McCammon, C. S.
1951   A study of four hundred seventy-five pregnancies in American Indian women. *American Journal of Obstetrics and Gynecology* 61: 1159—1166.
McDermott, W.
1966   Modern medicine and the demographic-disease pattern of overly traditional societies: a technologic misfit. *Journal of Medical Education* 4:137—162.
McDermott, W., K. Deuschle, J. Adair, H. Fulmer, and B. Loughlin
1960   Introducing modern medicine in a Navajo community. *Science* 131:197—205, 280—287.
McDermott, W., K. W. Deuschle, and C. R. Barnett
1972   Health care experiment at Many Farms. *Science* 175:23--31.
McFee, J. G.
1973   Anemia, a high risk complication of pregnancy. *Clinical Obstetrics and Gynecology* 16:153—171.
McKenzie, T.
1974   Testimony before the Permanent Subcommittee on Investigations of the Committee on Government Operations, U.S. Senate, 93rd Congress, 2d Session. Washington, D.C.: U.S. Government Printing Office.
McKeown, T.
1976a *The Modern Rise of Population.* New York: Academic Press, Inc.
1976b *The Role of Medicine.* London: The Nuffield Provincial Hospitals Trust.
McKinlay, J. B.
1975   The help-seeking behavior of the poor. In *Poverty and Health: A Sociological Analysis,* ed. J. Kosa and I. K. Zola, revised edition. Cambridge, Mass.: Harvard University Press.
May, P. A., and D. W. Broudy
n.d.   *Health Problems of the Navajo Area and Suggested Interventions,* 2d edition. Window Rock, Arizona: Navajo Health Authority.
May, P. A., D. W. Broudy, M. Yellowhair, K. Battese, and M. Hudson.
1977   Final Report: Comparative Health Services Evaluation Project, 1976—1977. Submitted to the Navajo Area Indian Health Service by the Navajo Health Authority, Window Rock, Arizona.
Menzel, H.
1950   Comment on Robinson's "Ecological correlations" and the behavior of individuals. *American Sociological Review* 15:674.
Meriam, L., and others.
1928   *The Problem of Indian Administration.* Institute for Government Research. Baltimore: The Johns Hopkins Press.
Moorman, L. J.
1949   Health of the Navajo-Hopi Indians, *Journal of the American Medical*

Association 139:370–376.

Morgan, K.
  1973 Historical demography of a Navajo community. In *Methods and Theories of Anthropological Genetics*, ed. M. H. Crawford and P. L. Workman. Albuquerque: University of New Mexico Press.

Morse, D.
  1961 Prehistoric tuberculosis in America. *American Review of Respiratory Diseases* 83:489–504.

Mountin, J. W., and J. G. Townsend
  1936 Observations on Indian Health Problems and Facilities. Public Health Bulletin no. 223. Washington, D.C.: U.S. Government Printing Office.

Murdock, G. P.
  1967 *Ethnographic Atlas*. Pittsburgh: University of Pittsburgh Press.

Navajo Area Indian Health Service
  1979a History of PL 86-121 funding on the Navajo Reservation. Unpublished data. Navajo Area Indian Health Service, U.S. Public Health Service, Window Rock, Arizona.
  1979b *Navajo Area Work Load and Notifiable Diseases*. Navajo Area Indian Health Service, U.S. Public Health Service, Window Rock, Arizona.

Navajo Health Systems Agency, Window Rock Arizona
  1978 *Navajo Health Systems Plan, 1978–1982*.

Navajo Medical News
  1940 Vols. 7 and 8, various issues. Medical Division, Navajo Service, Window Rock, Arizona. (Available from the National Archives, Washington, D.C.)

Navajo Times
  1978 The Morman Church in Navajoland. July 27:A2–4.

Navajo Tribe
  1968 *Navajo Manpower Survey*. Window Rock, Arizona.
  1974 *The Navajo Nation Overall Economic Development Program*. Window Rock, Arizona: Office of Program Development.

Nelson, B. D., J. Porvanznik, and J. R. Benfield
  1971 Gallbladder disease in southwestern American Indians. *Archives of Surgery* 103:41–43.

Neutra, R., J. E. Levy, and D. Parker
  1977 Cultural expectations versus reality in Navajo seizure patterns and sick roles. *Culture, Medicine and Society* 1:255–275.

North, C., T. Vollmer, and M. Goodwin
  1980 Obstetrical outcome in a remote first level care hospital serving Hopi and Navajo Indians. Paper presented at the 15th annual professional association meeting of the U.S. Public Health Service, May 26–29, Houston, Texas.

Oakland, L., and R. L. Kane
  1973 The working mother and child neglect on the Navajo reservation. *Pediatrics* 51:849–853.

Omran, A. R.
    1971   The epidemiologic transition: a theory of the epidemiology of population change. *The Milbank Memorial Fund Quarterly* 49: 509—538.
    1977   A century of epidemiologic transition in the U.S. *Preventive Medicine* 6:30—57.
Omran, A. R., and B. Loughlin
    1972   An epidemiologic study of accidents among the Navajo Indians. *The Journal of the Egyptian Medical Association* 55:1—22.
Page, I. H., L. A. Lewis, and J. Gilbert
    1956   Plasma lipids and proteins and their relationship to coronary disease among Navajo Indians. *Circulation* 13:675—679.
Parman, D. L.
    1976   *The Navajos and the New Deal.* New Haven: Yale University Press.
Paul, J. R., and G. L. Dixon
    1937   Climate and rheumatic disease. *Journal of the American Medical Association* 103:2096—2100.
Phelps-Stokes Fund
    1939   *The Navajo Indian Problem.* New York: The Phelps-Stokes Fund.
Philp, K. R.
    1977   *John Collier's Crusade for Indian Reform, 1920—1954.* Tucson: University of Arizona Press.
Pijoan, M., and McCammon, C. S.
    1949   The problem of medical care for Navajo Indians. *Journal of the American Medical Association* 140:1013—1949.
Pless, I. B.
    1974   The changing face of primary pediatrics. *Pediatric Clinics of North America* 21:223—244.
Polgar, S.
    1972   Population history and population policies from an anthropological perspective. *Current Anthropology* 13:203—211.
Preston, S. H.
    1976   *Mortality Patterns in National Populations.* New York: Academic Press, Inc.
Prosnitz, L. R., and E. E. Wallach
    1967   Unusual features of postpartum hypopituitarism among American Indians of the Southwest. *Obstetrics and Gynecology* 29: 351—357.
Reagan, A. B.
    1919   The influenza and the Navajo. *Proceedings of the Indiana Academy of Science* 29:243—247.
Reichard, G. A.
    1963   *Navajo Religion*, 2d edition. New York: Pantheon Books.
Reifel, A.
    1949   Tuberculosis among Indians of the United States. *Diseases of the Chest* 16:234—247.
Reisinger, K. K., D. Rogers, and O. Johnson

1972   Nutritional survey of lower Greasewood, Arizona Navajos. In *Nutrition, Growth and Development of North American Indian Children*, ed. W. M. Moore, M. M. Silverberg, and M. S. Read. DHEW Publication no. (NIH) 72–76. Washington, D.C.: U.S. Government Printing Office.

Reno, P.
1970   Manpower planning for Navajo employment: training for jobs in a surplus-labor area. *New Mexico Business* (Nov–Dec): 8–16.

Robbins, L.
1975   *The Impact of Industrial Developments on the Navajo Nation*. Bulletin 7, Lake Powell Research Project. Los Angeles: Institute of Geophysics and Planetary Physics, University of California.

Robinson, W. S.
1950   Ecological correlations and the behavior of individuals. *American Sociological Review* 15:351–357.

Rogers, K. D., R. Ernst, I. Shulman, and K. Reisinger
1974   Effectiveness of aggressive follow-up on Navajo infant health and medical care use. *Pediatrics* 53:721–725.

Rubenstein, A., J. Boyle, C. L. Odoroff, and S. J. Kunitz
1969   Effect of improved sanitary facilities on infant diarrhea in a Hopi village. *Public Health Reports* 84:1093–1097.

Ruffing, L. T.
1974   *Alternative Economic Development Policies for Indian Communities: Economic Development and Navajo Social Structure*. U.S. Department of Commerce, Economic Development Administration, Office of Economic Research. Washington, D.C.

Safran, N.
1940   Infant Mortality. *Navajo Medical News* 7, no. 1: 13–15. Window Rock, Arizona: BIA Navajo Medical Service.

Sampliner, R. E., P. H. Bennett, L. J. Comess, F. A. Rose, and T. A. Burch
1970   Gallbladder disease in Pima Indians: demonstration of prevalence and early onset by cholecystography. *New England Journal of Medicine* 283:1358–1364.

Savishinsky, J. S.
1971   Mobility as an aspect of stress in an arctic community. *American Anthropologist* 73:604–618.

Schnur, L.
1942   Navajos train ward aides to counteract "medicine man." *The Modern Hospital* 59:80.

Scrimshaw, N., C. E. Taylor, and J. E. Gordon
1959   Interactions of nutrition and infection. *American Journal of Medical Science* 237:367–403.

Secretary of the Treasury
1913   Contagious and Infectious Diseases among the Indians. Report to the Committee on Indian Affairs, 63rd Congress, 3rd Session, Senate Document No. 1038. Washington, D.C.: U.S. Government Printing Office.

Seldin, D. W.

1975 The intimate coupling of biomedical science and physician education. *Clinical Research* 23:280–286.

1976 Specialization as scientific advancement and overspecialization as
social distortion. *Clinical Research* 24:245–248.

Selye, Hans

1956 *The Stress of Life.* New York: McGraw-Hill Book Company, Inc.

Shepardson, M.

1982 Changing attitudes towards Navajo religion. In *Navajo Religion and
Culture: Selected Views.* Papers in honor of Leland C.Wyman, ed.
D. M. Brugge and C. J. Frisbie. Santa Fe: Museum of New Mexico
Press.

Shepardson, M., and B. Hammond

1964 Change and persistence in an isolated Navajo community. *American
Anthropologist* 66:1029–1049.

Sievers, M. L.

1967 Myocardial infarction among southwestern American Indians. *Annals of Internal Medicine* 67:800–807.

1968 Cigarette and alcohol usage by southwestern American Indians.
American Journal of Public Health 58:71–82.

Sievers, M. L., and J. R. Marquis

1962 The southwestern Indian's burden: biliary diseases. *Journal of the
American Medical Association* 182:172–174.

Slocumb, J. C., and S. J. Kunitz

1977 Factors affecting maternal mortality and morbidity among American Indians. *Public Health Reports* 92:349–356.

Slocumb, J. C., S. J. Kunitz, and C. L. Odoroff

1979 Complications with use of IUD and oral contraceptives among
Navajo women. *Public Health Reports* 94:243–247.

Slocumb, J. C., C. L. Odoroff, and S. J. Kunitz

1975 The use-effectiveness of two contraceptive methods in a Navajo
population: the problem of program dropouts. *American Journal of
Obstetrics and Gynecology* 122:717–726.

Small, D. M., and S. Rapo

1970 Source of abnormal bile in patients with cholesterol gallstones. *New
England Journal of Medicine* 283:53–57.

Smith, R. L.

1957 Cardio-vascular-renal and diabetes deaths among the Navajos.
Public Health Reports 72:33–38.

Snedecor, G. W., and W. G. Cochran

1967 *Statistical Methods.* Ames, Iowa: Iowa State University Press.

Sorkin, A. L.

1971 *American Indians and Federal Aid.* Washington, D.C.: The Brookings
Institution.

Spicer, E. H.

1961 Types of contact and processes of change. In *Perspectives in American Indian Cultural Change*, ed. E. H. Spicer. Chicago: University of
Chicago Press.

Stewart, T., P. May, and A. Muneta
1980   A Navajo health consumer survey. *Medical Care* 18:1183–1195.
Streeper, R. B., R. U. Massey, G. Liu, C. H. Dillingham, and A. Cushing
1960   An electrocardiographic and autopsy study of coronary heart disease in the Navajo. *Diseases of the Chest* 38:305–312.
Temkin-Greener, H., S. J. Kunitz, D. Broudy, and M. Haffner
1981   Surgical fertility regulation among women on the Navajo Indian reservation, 1972–1978. *American Journal of Public Health* 71: 403–407.
Thistle, J. L., K. L. Eckhart, R. E. Nensel, F. T. Nobrega, G. G. Poehling, M. Reimer, and L. J. Schoenfield
1971   Prevalence of gallbladder disease among Chippewa Indians. *Mayo Clinic Proceedings.* 46:603–608.
Thompson, L.
1951   *Personality and Government.* Mexico, D.F.: Ediciones del Instituto Indigenista Interamericano.
Thompson, L., and A. Joseph
1947   *The Hopi Way.* Chicago: University of Chicago Press.
Tillim, S. J.
1936   Health among the Navajos. *Southwestern Medicine* 20:355, 388, 432.
TNY
1958   The Navajo Yearbook. Window Rock, Arizona: Bureau of Indian Affairs.
1961   The Navajo Yearbook. Window Rock, Arizona: Bureau of Indian Affairs.
Trowell, H. C., and D. P. Burkitt
1981   *Western Diseases: Their Emergence and Prevention.* London: Edward Arnold.
Underhill, R. M.
1948   *Ceremonial Patterns in the Greater Southwest.* Monographs of the American Ethnological Society, no. 13. Seattle: University of Washington Press.
1963   *The Navajos.* Norman: University of Oklahoma Press.
United Nations
1965   *Population Bulletin,* no. 7 (ST/SOA/ser. N.). New York.
U.S. Bureau of the Census
1972   *Census of Population, 1970.* U.S. Summary, General Population Characteristics PC (1)-B1. Washington, D.C.: U.S. Government Printing Office.
1973   *Census of Population, 1970.* Subject Report PC(2)-1F, American Indians. Washington, D.C.: U.S. Government Printing Office.
1977   *Reports on the findings of special enumeration-population register match for three chapter of Navajo Reservation.* Washington, D.C.: U.S. Government Printing Office.
U.S. Bureau of Indian Affairs
1973   *Estimates of resident Indian population and labor force status; by state and reservation: March 1973.* Washington, D.C.: Department of the Interior.

U.S. Public Health Service
    1957   *Health Services for American Indians.* U.S. Department of Health,
            Education and Welfare, PHS Publication no. 531. Washington,
            D.C.: Government Printing Office.
    1959   *The Indian Health Program from 1800–1955.* Washington, D.C.:
            Department of Health, Education and Welfare. Public Health
            Service, Division of Indian Health.
    1970a   *1968 Indian Vital Statistics, Navajo Area.* Indian Health Service,
            Health Program Systems Center, Tucson, Arizona.
    1970b   *Indian Vital Statistics C.Y. 1969.* Indian Health Service, Health Pro-
            gram Systems Center, Tucson, Arizona.
    1971   *Indian Health Trends and Services,* 1970 edition. PHS Publication
            no. 2092. Washington, D.C.: Indian Health Service, Office of Pro-
            gram Planning and Evaluation, Program Analysis and Statistics
            Branch.
    1973   *Ambulatory patient care services, Injuries.* Window Rock, Arizona:
            Navajo Area Office, Indian Health Service.
    1979   *Selected Vital Statistics for Indian Health Service Areas and Service Units,
            1972–1977.* DHEW Publication no. (HSA) 79–1005. Washing-
            ton, D.C.

U.S. Soil Conservation Service
    1939   *Statistical Summary: Human Dependency Survey, Navajo and Hopi Res-
            ervations.* Section of Conservation Economics, Navajo Area, Re-
            gion 8, Aug. 8, 1938, revised May, 1939.

Van Duzen, J., J. P. Carter, J. Secondi, and C. Federspiel
    1969   Protein and calorie malnutrition among pre-school Navajo Indian
            children. *The American Journal of Clinical Nutrition* 22:1362–1370.

Vaughn, J. B.
    1969   Maternal deaths in New Mexico, 1956–1966. *Rocky Mountain
            Medical Journal* 66:65–70.

Vogt, E. Z.
    1951   *Navajo Veterans, a Study of Changing Values.* Cambridge, Mass.:
            Peabody Museum, Harvard University.
    1961   Navajo. In *Perspectives in American Indian Culture Change,* ed. E. H.
            Spicer. Chicago: University of Chicago Press.

Wallach, E. E., A. E. Beer, and C.-R. Garcia
    1967   Patient acceptance of oral contraceptives, 1. The American Indian.
            American Journal of Obstetrics and Gynecology 97:984–991.

Werner, O.
    1965   Semantics of Navajo medical terms: I. *International Journal of
            American Linguistics* 31:1–17.

White, K. L., D. O. Anderson, T. W. Bice, and E. Schah
    1976   Health care: an international comparison of perceived morbidity,
            health services resources and use. *International Journal of Health
            Services* 6:199–218.

Wistisen, M. J., R. J. Parsons, and A. Larsen
    1975   *A Study to Identify Potentially Feasible Small Businesses for the Navajo.*

Provo, Utah: Center for Business and Economic Research, Survey Research Center, Brigham Young University.

Wolf, C. B.
  1961   Kwashiorkor on the Navajo Indian reservation. *Henry Ford Hospital Medical Bulletin* 9:566–571.

Woods, O. T.
  1947   Health among the Navajo Indians. *Journal of the American Medical Association* 135:981–983.

Wyman, L. C.
  1936   Origin legend of Navajo divinatory rites. *Journal of American Folklore* 49:134–142.

Wyman, L. C., and F. L. Bailey
  1964   *Navajo Indian Enthnoentomology*. Albuquerque: University of New Mexico Press.

Wyman, L. C., and S. K. Harris
  1951   *The Ethnobotany of the Kayenta Navaho*. Albuquerque: University of New Mexico Publications in Biology 5.

Wyman, L. C., and C. Kluckhohn
  1938   *Navajo Classification of Their Song Ceremonials*. American Anthropological Association Memoir, 50.

York, R. J.
  1979   *The Continuum of Life: Health Concerns of the Indian Elderly*. Albuquerque: Indian Council on Aging.

Index

Designer:	UC Press Staff
Compositor:	Trend Western
Text:	Baskerville 11/13
Display:	Baskerville
Printer:	Maple-Vail Book Mfg. Group
Binder:	Maple-Vail Book Mfg. Group